The Psychosocial Impact of Rheumatic Conditions

Jillian Rose-Smith • Melissa Flores
Priscilla Calvache

The Psychosocial Impact of Rheumatic Conditions

Caring for the Whole Patient

Springer

Jillian Rose-Smith
Hospital for Special Surgery
New York, NY, USA

Melissa Flores
Hospital for Special Surgery
New York, NY, USA

Priscilla Calvache
Hospital for Special Surgery
New York, NY, USA

ISBN 978-3-031-95337-8 ISBN 978-3-031-95338-5 (eBook)
https://doi.org/10.1007/978-3-031-95338-5

This Springer imprint is published by the registered company Springer Nature Switzerland AG
The registered company address is: Gewerbestrasse 11, 6330 Cham, Switzerland

This book is dedicated to the longstanding work and incredible career of Roberta Horton, LCSW, ACSW, who served as a compassionate leader, educator, and mentor to each of us in our social work careers. We would also like to dedicate this book to all the patients who have allowed us to walk side by side with them on their journey. May their courage, resilience, and hope inspire others, just as they inspire us every day.

Foreword

It is a privilege to introduce this important book because of the impact I know it will have on the community of patients living with chronic rheumatic diseases. As a patient with lupus for over 50 years, I am thrilled to endorse a resource for a population of patients who face unique and unpredictable symptoms, which often have no answers to why, where, or when it rears its ugly head.

I have had the fortunate experience of working with all three authors through Hospital for Special Surgery's exceptional support and education programs for patients with rheumatic illnesses for over 15 years as both a patient and volunteer. Their commitment to patients and their loved ones, their innovative programs that leverage the peer support model, their intentionality in galvanizing the interdisciplinary team, strengthening the doctor-patient partnership, and their values for inclusivity, diversity, and community outreach have inspired me to continue to support their ever-evolving projects.

As a volunteer, I was invited to write a book for children with lupus, addressing the unique challenges faced by the pediatric populations and their families. This book focused on educating children about the symptoms of lupus, empowering them to share their illness with friends and family highlighting that lupus does not define who they are. Several thousand copies of this resource were disseminated to pediatric rheumatology hospitals across the country. Their goal is to provide a resource for not only the children but their parents and the physicians who care for them.

Additionally, I provide weekly counseling over the phone to people with lupus and their loved ones and support with the ongoing training of peer volunteers.

The contents of this book reflect the essentials of working with the whole patient, as living with an unpredictable chronic illness has its own set of challenges. There is special difficulty knowing that your days of pain and ever-changing indicators are uncertain and unknown. The feeling of a lifetime of roadblocks must be addressed by the caregivers and medical team. It is critical to assess and address the psychosocial impact of their illness to best support the patient holistically. Through this book rheumatology providers and allied health professionals will be equipped with a unique resource to guide and support the care that they provide to patients living with rheumatic illness.

Judith Campbell MS in counseling; was on President Obama's Health Committee in 2008; co-authored "Variance in treatment and costs by antidepressant class: Analysis in an HMO" in FORMULARY, March 2001. Vol. 36, No. 3; and was formerly the Director of Alliance Development for Pfizer Inc

Judith Campbell

Preface

"Get to know the entire person—their whole humanity versus just who they are as a patient." These were words from a woman with systemic lupus erythematosus (SLE) when asked about her patient journey and what she would like providers to consider when treating patients with rheumatic illness.

As social workers and public health professionals, we have walked alongside people impacted by rheumatic illness—laughed with, cried with, advocated, but most importantly, listened—for patients are the experts of their own lives. We have made it our mission to meet patients where they are and elevate their voices to get the care they deserve. By applying a social work lens, this book delves into the complexities of treating not just the illness itself but the whole person. In this book we share the work we have been immersed in for the past two decades. This book provides the tools and strategies that we have applied in our work with patients and providers, while told through patient stories—and highlighting model programs. We invite you to learn them, use them, and together we can provide much-needed, comprehensive care to the *whole* patient.

New York, NY, USA Jillian Rose-Smith
New York, NY, USA Melissa Flores
New York, NY, USA Priscilla Calvache

Acknowledgments

We are profoundly grateful to our families—especially our partners, Eon, Andres, and Steve—for their unwavering support throughout our journey of writing this book. And to our children, Bellarose, Aking, Isabella, and Amelia, who constantly remind us of what truly matters and inspire us to leave the world better than we found it.

Contents

1 **Introduction: The Rheumatology Patient Journey** 1

2 **Psychosocial Aspects of Rheumatic Conditions** 3

3 **Tools for Addressing Psycho-Social-Emotional Aspects of Care** 15

4 **The Patient-Provider Partnership: It's a Dance!** . . . 21

5 **Cultural Considerations and Addressing Patient Values** 37

6 **Special Populations in Rheumatology: LGBTQIA+ Identity** 47

7 **Navigating the Path to Adherence: Fostering Collaborative Patient-Centered Care** 61

8 **Using a Team Approach to Achieve Optimal Outcomes** 73

9 **Engaging the Family and Support System in Patient Care** 87

10 **Self-Management and Patient Education Interventions** 97

11 **Health Disparities and Confronting Implicit Bias as a Strategy to Address Them** 109

12 **Beyond the Exam Room: Addressing Social Determinants of Health** 121

13 **The Impact of a Global Health Pandemic, Telehealth, and the Digital Divide** 139

14 **Engaging Patients in Research: Incorporating the Patient Perspective**. 151

Index. 165

Introduction: The Rheumatology Patient Journey

1

Patients and their loved ones enter the patient journey at various points and with differing circumstances, presentations, and emotional and psychological states. They bring with them a unique set of lived experiences and different lenses in which they view health, well-being, and healthcare. Many with rheumatic illnesses are thrust into a vortex of unexplained symptoms, with no clear explanation of the cause, and are forced to traverse between different specialists and health systems only to find no clear answers for their symptoms and the betrayal of their bodies. Others come into the journey based on a history and evidence of rheumatic illness in their families. However, despite seeing and experiencing others living their lives with a chronic rheumatic illness, the journey is different for each individual and can be riddled with different pain points, successes, and challenges. Yet, others come in by accidental findings, only experiencing subtle changes in form and function that cause minimal disruption to their lives. No matter the portal of entry, patients traversing this journey need clinicians and care teams to understand them as whole individuals, building meaningful, trust-based relationships that serve as pathways to quality care and, ultimately, optimal outcomes.

There is much for us to consider as care providers and navigators of this journey for patients who are often confused and scared of the unknown trajectory of their conditions. How can we be best prepared to treat and manage a diverse group of patients who

J. Rose-Smith et al., *The Psychosocial Impact of Rheumatic Conditions*, https://doi.org/10.1007/978-3-031-95338-5_1

often present with complex illnesses as well as complex life situations? To create mutually beneficial therapeutic relationships that allow us to understand and treat the whole person successfully, it's important that we consider what is valuable to the patient, using techniques to create partnerships and engage the patient voice in care. We should seek to understand the lived environment of the patient and how where they live, work, and play can impact their illness and treatment recommendations. Cultural considerations are key to successfully managing patients on this journey, and checking our own biases can help us better understand our patients and treat them with empathy, dignity, and respect. Using a team approach that includes the patient, their loved ones, and the interprofessional team has also been proven to enhance quality and optimize care for this population. Using key tools and strategies to assess and address the psychosocial realities of patients and integrating that information into creating appropriate treatment plans can optimize adherence and self-management. This book provides key information and strategies to support the rheumatic care provider in managing the psychosocial impact of a rheumatic illness on patients and demonstrates how to successfully engage them as care partners for the best outcomes, experience, and satisfaction on this journey.

Psychosocial Aspects of Rheumatic Conditions

2

Rheumatic conditions can have major effects on all aspects of a person's life. Regardless of the severity level of the condition, people living with rheumatic conditions will need to manage both emotional and physical symptoms. For example, patients living with systemic lupus erythematosus (SLE) often cope with daily pain, fatigue, and mobility limitations. The unpredictability and uncertainty that often characterize rheumatic conditions can also affect a person's ability to manage stress, activities of daily living, and social and professional obligations.

Mourning Your Old Self: Loss and Grief When Living with a Rheumatic Condition

Rheumatic conditions are often unpredictable and may cause significant lifestyle changes. There are psychosocial challenges, such as feelings of isolation due to the invisible nature of the illness, and physical and cognitive manifestations. People may react to the news of a new diagnosis with a variety of emotions, such as shock, fear, stress, or anger. Some may go from seeing a physician once a year to multiple specialists monthly with a new regimen of daily medications. Issues concerning one's identity as a partner, spouse, or parent may come into question and impact a person's self-esteem [1].

J. Rose-Smith et al., *The Psychosocial Impact of Rheumatic Conditions*, https://doi.org/10.1007/978-3-031-95338-5_2

These life changes are inevitably accompanied by a sense of loss and grief. Grief is a very normal reaction to the loss of one's physical health from prior to their diagnosis and beyond. As healthcare professionals, it is critical to acknowledge the grieving process with which people living with rheumatic conditions must often cope. There is a process of mourning their past self or their sense of identity pre-diagnosis. Patients often describe feeling like their body has betrayed them, leaving them feeling "out of control." Others feel that their life dramatically shifted from one day to the next due to significant changes to work, hobbies, and interests that often formed a person's identity. There are fears around one's mortality and ability to care for themselves, children, and loved ones. People may be dealing with multiple losses, such as friends, work, and personal relationships, in addition to their physical health.

The Five Stages of Grief, coined by Elisabeth Kubler-Ross, include denial, anger, depression, bargaining, and acceptance. This widely cited model is a helpful framework to help patients process, and providers to explain, the feelings of grief or loss of their "old life" before their rheumatic condition diagnosis. Recognizing this sense of loss can help patients work through many complex emotions discussed above. In a chronic illness, the grieving process is cyclical. Like the illness itself, however, it does not necessarily follow a linear progression, making it impossible to predict the stages patients will experience as they cope with different aspects of their condition [2].

The stages of grief can actually have both positive and negative sides to them. They are positive when they help clients cope with their loss. They are negative to the extent that they hinder the client's ability to prosper or function. Additionally, a person's way of adapting to previous life challenges before developing a rheumatic condition, family, culture, gender roles, and available support systems all influence the grieving process.

When treating some of the physical manifestations of rheumatic conditions, it's equally important to discuss the many lifestyle changes and the emotional toll they may take on the patient. Research has demonstrated the power of the patient-doctor relationship. We know that physician behaviors and attitudes can have a considerable impact on relationship-building and developing trust with patients, leading to better overall health outcomes.

Impact on Relationships and Social Roles

Each person's experience with their condition is different, including their comfort level in sharing this part of their life. It is normal for patients to experience a range of emotions when considering whether and how much to disclose about their condition—whether with loved ones, at school or work, or even with their healthcare team.

The many misconceptions about a rheumatic condition and the invisibility of the disease itself may sometimes cause patients to feel isolated and stigmatized by others. When you do not fit the image of what a "sick person" looks like, those around you may struggle to understand the person's experience with symptoms like fatigue and physical and emotional pain. Patients often describe difficulties with keeping social commitments and continuing to work. Some patients may delay sharing significant symptoms with their healthcare provider and often struggle to explain their condition to family or loved ones. For some, this is due to a desire to appear "normal" and to minimize feeling like they are always complaining about their symptoms, conditions, and life changes [3, 4].

Although it can be daunting for patients to reveal the full extent of their illness, doing so fosters a critical connection with their support system and healthcare team, helping them to optimize other areas of their emotional well-being, such as self-esteem and mood.

Often providers find themselves challenged by how to address these concerns during the medical visit. Connecting with other interdisciplinary members of the healthcare team, such as social workers and nurse colleagues, is important to support patients in addressing work and relationship concerns. Openly asking patients to reflect on the following questions: *What am I most concerned about in talking about my rheumatic condition? What can I gain, and what might I have to lose when disclosing to others?* Answers to these questions can support open communication and trust around these concerns. The discussion will help patients identify the level of risk they are willing to take when sharing with colleagues, friends, loved ones, and their healthcare team. A few other helpful reminders for rheumatology health professionals include the following:

- If patients are having trouble explaining physical symptoms or information about their condition, consider asking them to invite a loved one to a medical visit, support group, or educational workshop. This may help the patient understand more about the condition and how it not only affects them but also their loved ones.
- Remind patients that they are in control of what and how much information they share about their condition with others. They should never feel pressured to disclose more than they are comfortable with.
- Invite conversations around patient cultural norms, values, and health practices and how they may affect the management of their condition. Personal health beliefs can affect how they make decisions about everything from discussing symptoms to medications and treatment plans.
- Ask patients how their rheumatic condition is impacting them both physically and emotionally. Fostering open communication will help to build trust. Remember to validate feelings and experiences. It can take a while for patients to feel comfortable enough to talk with others about their condition. Being connected to a mental health professional who is familiar with rheumatic conditions or chronic illness may also be helpful in getting your patient the right support and building new coping strategies.
- Refer patients to a responsible chronic illness or disease-specific community to feel less alone—either online, by phone, or in person. These communities may impart strategies to manage one's illness and a platform for sharing experiences that can assist patients in coping with a rheumatic condition.

Navigating Work Accommodations

Rheumatic conditions can result in significant changes to work roles, including changes to work responsibilities, transitioning to part-time work, disability, or early retirement [5]. Patients often rely on and seek direct guidance from their medical providers on how to best navigate changes in work, request reasonable accommodations, or apply for temporary or permanent disability [6].

In general, it is encouraged that patients plan to disclose a disability when they are looking to request a reasonable accommodation, such as an ergonomic chair or special lighting to assist with photosensitivity issues or even a schedule change. Many people with invisible medical conditions like lupus, rheumatoid arthritis (RA), and other rheumatic illness may feel that they are not being completely honest with an employer if they do not tell everything about their disability upfront at the time of their interview. Patients are not obligated to do so. When disclosing a medical condition, a general rule is to provide basic information about the condition, its limitations, and the accommodations they may need. It is also helpful to consider the timing of when to disclose their condition; patients may not want to wait until they begin to experience work performance issues. It is often better to disclose your disability and request an accommodation before job performance is impacted or conduct problems occur. Remember, the purpose of an accommodation is to enable a qualified person with a disability to perform the essential functions of the job. So, it may be helpful for patients to disclose when they first realize they are having difficulties.

Sex and Intimacy

Sex and intimacy are often complex subjects to discuss openly for both patients and providers. However, it's important to address these issues for patients to maintain a satisfying sex life and healthy intimate relationships. This subject may be particularly tense for those living with systemic lupus erythematosus, or lupus. Studies suggest people with lupus often abstain from sexual activity and avoid intimate relationships for a variety of reasons, including side effects of medication, mood changes, and physical challenges. All of these can affect sexual function, desire, and behavior in both women and men with lupus [7].

Some people have been known to reduce their engagement in sexual relations when faced with challenging medical symptoms. In some women, physical effects of the disease may include limited range of motion in the hips or knees and decreased vaginal lubrication. Men are reported to have higher rates of impotence. Chronic pain, stiffness, and fatigue, as well as certain medications, may also decrease sexual desire among people with lupus [8].

Often issues regarding sexual dysfunction and intimacy issues remain unaddressed in the medical setting. "Poor communication between physicians and patients is the most likely explanation, along with poor communication between patients and their partners. However, the reasons for this communication gap, which may range from stigma to time constraints in the clinic, are up for debate" [9].

Research shows that the lack of optimal doctor-patient communication can contribute to miscommunication or lack of trust in the medical setting. Further negatively confounding issues often at play in the doctor-patient relationship include language barriers, cultural beliefs and values, and implicit bias [10]. Patients want to talk about sexual intimacy concerns but may shy away due to embarrassment or shame. Strong communication between the patient and provider can help to minimize the challenges of bringing up these sensitive topics. Preparing some strong open-ended questions to understand the impact of the illness on this area of care can help to start these conversations in the medical setting and build trust over time. For example:

- To what extent have you experienced any changes in your sexual/intimate desire/interest?
- How is your condition impacting your sexual function right now?
- Sex and intimacy are often an important part of our lives; tell me about how your illness is impacting this area.

- Has your condition impacted your intimate or sexual relationship with your partner?
- Have you spoken with your doctor regarding concerns you may have about your reproductive health?
- Due to the impact of your condition, are you concerned about your ability to have children?

Mental Health Considerations

Disparities lie in the availability, accessibility, and quality of mental health services, and some ethnic groups are impacted at higher rates by poor mental health outcomes. Additionally, people who have a history of depression and/or stressful events leading up to diagnosis may have an increased risk of experiencing grief or psychological challenges when diagnosed with a chronic illness. According to the National Institute of Mental Health [11], people living with a chronic illness, like autoimmune diseases, including systemic lupus erythematosus or rheumatoid arthritis, may be more likely to be impacted by depression.

For example, depression can occur as a reaction to some of the daily challenges of adjusting to living with a chronic illness, or as a result of the newly prescribed medication and/or treatment plan. In SLE, clinical depression may not be easily recognized because its symptoms are similar to those of SLE. For example, lack of energy and trouble sleeping can be attributed to the condition itself. However, these are also symptoms of clinical depression.

"Research has demonstrated that treating depression and the rheumatic condition at the same time can help patients to better manage both their mental health and chronic condition" [11]. For many, the topic of mental health is often taboo. Patients may feel concerned that if they open up about mental health concerns, it will lead to poor public perception by their loved ones, friends, or even their healthcare team. Questions such as "Will people judge me or think I'm crazy?" make it harder to speak up and seek support. In many other cultures or religions, speaking about family or personal issues may be considered a sign of disrespect, weakness, and is highly discouraged. This is important to acknowledge because it affects how health beliefs are shaped and how patients may choose to manage stress, depression, and other mental health concerns.

As healthcare professionals, it's important to educate patients on the interconnection they may experience between their physical and emotional health. For some patients, it may be a challenge to understand the mind-body connection. This means that our thoughts, feelings, beliefs, and attitudes can positively or negatively affect our biological functioning. In other words, our minds can affect our physical health [12]. As healthcare providers, we should underscore that caring for our mental health is just as important as our physical health. A helpful example is looking at how we manage our physical health, the same way we would seek care for a broken bone; it is important to seek care when you are noticing your thoughts, mood, or overall emotions are affecting your day-to-day life.

For example, studies show that mindfulness-based practices improve our ability to cope with conditions such as anxiety. Just 10 min of quiet reflection, deep breathing, or guided imagery may bring relief from stress and can increase one's tolerance for it. A study that examined the effect of mindfulness-based stress reduction (MBSR) in rheumatoid arthritis (RA) patients saw a positive "change in depressive symptoms, with secondary outcomes of change in psychological distress, well-being, mindfulness, and RA disease activity" for patients who had a regular MBSR practice for 6 months [13, 14].

Depression and Anxiety in Rheumatic Conditions

Research shows that chronic illness can have a profound impact on a person's psychosocial well-being. Chronic illness is consistently associated with depression and anxiety, as found in numerous studies. For example, people with lupus and RA often report feelings of isolation due to characteristics of the disease, feelings of grief, loss, and difficulty coping with uncertainty. Research also tells us that patients with support cope better with their condition and are less likely to experience these challenges [15].

Depression and anxiety disorders are both mental health conditions. They each have their own causes, emotional, and behavioral symptoms. Being aware of the risks and warning signs is an essential component of supporting the overall psychosocial health of patients. In rheumatic conditions, untreated depression and anxiety can have a detrimental impact on the overall management of conditions, such as forgetting or stopping taking medications, decreased follow-up with medical providers, and more. If one is already coping with depression or anxiety, new stressors may exacerbate or make one's ability to manage their current symptoms even more challenging [16].

It is important to understand the difference between feelings of *sadness* and *clinical depression*. Feelings of sadness tend to come and go and may be related to something going on in your life. Usually, this sadness does not affect your ability to function for any length of time. To be diagnosed with clinical depression, symptoms must persist for 2 weeks or longer and represent a significant change from previous functioning [17].

The most common form of depression diagnosed is major depression. Some of the warning signs include:

- Feeling a lack of energy.
- Overeating or under-eating.
- Inability to sleep or excessive sleeping.
- Increase alcohol and drug consumption as a way of coping.
- Feelings of worthlessness or excessive guilt.
- Recurrent thoughts of death and suicidal ideation and other cognitive difficulties.

Similar to depression, it is normal for patients to feel some sort of anxiety in relation to life stressors and coping with a chronic condition. While this type of anxiety is unpleasant, it often motivates all of us to strive for success or put in our best effort. In the case of an anxiety disorder, the feeling of fear may be with you all the time. It is intense and sometimes debilitating and may cause you to stop doing things you enjoy. There are several forms of anxiety-related conditions, and the most common form of anxiety is called generalized anxiety disorder. The main symptom of anxiety disorders is excessive fear or worry. Your specific symptoms depend on the type of anxiety disorder you have.

Common anxiety symptoms also include:

- Panic and fear.
- Uneasiness.
- Sleep problems.
- Not being able to find a sense of calm and still.

Some physical symptoms include feeling cold, sweaty, numb, or tingling hands or feet, shortness of breath, breathing faster and more quickly than normal (hyperventilation), heart palpitations, or rumination—when you think about a problem repeatedly and are unable to stop.

Being familiar with the risks and warning signs of these mental health conditions can support rheumatology professionals in supporting patients impacted by depression and anxiety. If you notice your patient experiencing major changes in their overall functioning—for example, they start missing work or school or stop going to classes, medical appointments, or other usual social activities—these are important red flags. This is when we want to pay more attention to these symptoms and reach out for additional support from social work colleagues or refer to community-based resources to help patients identify new ways of coping.

References

1. Sutanto B, Singh-Grewal D, McNeil HP, O'Neill S, Craig JC, Jones J, et al. Experiences and perspectives of adults living with systemic lupus erythematosus: thematic synthesis of qualitative studies. Arthritis Care Res. 2013;65(11):1752–65.
2. Tyrrell P, Harberger S, Schoo C, Siddiqui W. Kubler-Ross stages of dying and subsequent models of grief. StatPearls. Treasure Island (FL): StatPearls Publishing Copyright © 2023, StatPearls Publishing LLC; 2023.
3. Mendelsohn S, Khoja L, Alfred S, He J, Anderson M, DuBois D, et al. Cognitive impairment in systemic lupus erythematosus is negatively

related to social role participation and quality of life: a systematic review. Lupus. 2021;30(10):1617–30.
4. Sayadi L, Faezi ST, Hasanpour M, Alahmadi SJ. The relationship of lifestyle with disease activity among patients with systemic lupus erythematosus: a descriptive-correlational study. Mediterr J Rheumatol. 2021;32(2):124–33.
5. Collins TR. Studies say people with rheumatic disease face work challenges: the rheumatologist. 2020. https://www.the-rheumatologist.org/article/studies-say-people-with-rheumatic-disease-face-work-challenges/. Accessed 21 Apr 2021.
6. Xiang L, Low AHL, Leung YY, Fong W, Gan WH, Graves N, et al. Work disability in rheumatic diseases: baseline results from an inception cohort. Int J Rheum Dis. 2020;23(8):1040–9.
7. Moghadam ZB, Rezaei E, Faezi ST, Zareian A, Ibrahim FM, Ibrahim MM. Prevalence of sexual dysfunction in women with systemic lupus erythematosus and its related factors. Reumatologia. 2019;57(1):19–26.
8. de Almeida PH, de Castro Ferreira C, Kurizky PS, Muniz LF, da Mota LM. How the rheumatologist can guide the patient with rheumatoid arthritis on sexual function. Rev Bras Reumatol. 2015;55:458–63.
9. Dikranian AH. Unspoken and undiagnosed: addressing sex and intimacy issues in rheumatic disease: Healio.com. 2017. https://www.healio.com/news/rheumatology/20170614/unspoken-and-undiagnosed-addressing-sex-and-intimacy-issues-in-rheumatic-disease. Accessed 21 Apr 2021.
10. Gynecologists ACoOa. Effective patient–physician communication. 2014. https://www.acog.org/clinical/clinical-guidance/committee-opinion/articles/2014/02/effective-patient-physician-communication#:~:text=Differences%20between%20physicians%20and%20patients,and%20gender%20can%20affect%20care. Accessed 21 Apr 2021.
11. Health NIoM. Chronic illness and mental health: recognizing and treating depression: U.S. Department of Health and Human Services, National Institutes of Health. 2021. https://www.nimh.nih.gov/health/publications/chronic-illness-mental-health. Accessed 21 April 2021.
12. Retzlaff K. Mind-body focus can improve treatment, outcomes in rheumatic disease: the rheumatologist. 2015. https://www.the-rheumatologist.org/article/mind-body-focus-can-improve-treatment-outcomes-in-rheumatic-disease/2/. Accessed 21 Apr 2021.
13. Schmehr LR. Mind-body practices for enhanced well-being when living with rheumatoid arthritis. New York: Hospital for Special Surgery; 2016. https://www.hss.edu/conditions_mind-body-practices-well-being-living-rheumatoid-arthritis.asp#references. Accessed 21 Apr 2021
14. Nguyen TT, Jensen CG, Khoury L, Deleuran B, Blom ES, Breinholt T, et al. Effectiveness of mind-body intervention for inflammatory conditions: results from a 26-week randomized, non-blinded, parallel-group trial. J Clin Med. 2021;10(14)

15. Peterson S, Piercy J, Blackburn S, Sullivan E, Karyekar CS, Li N. The multifaceted impact of anxiety and depression on patients with rheumatoid arthritis. BMC Rheumatol. 2019;3:43.
16. Beckerman NL, Auerbach C, Kim SJ, Salmon J, Horton R. Lupus (SLE): existence and impact of depressive symptomatology. Soc Work Health Care. 2015;54:499–517.
17. Prevention CfDCa. Mental health conditions: depression and anxiety: office on smoking and health, national center for chronic disease prevention and health promotion. 2022. [updated] September 14, 2022. https://www.cdc.gov/tobacco/campaign/tips/diseases/depression-anxiety.html. Accessed 21 Apr 2021.

Tools for Addressing Psycho-Social-Emotional Aspects of Care

3

Risk, Assessment, and Intervention

Living with a chronic illness is a risk factor that may lead to depression or suicide ideation. Studies have demonstrated that people with poor mental health, poor quality of life, low socioeconomic status, and limited family support were more vulnerable to depression and suicidal behaviors compared with other people [1].

Assessing for suicide risk is important, especially if healthcare providers begin to notice decline and major changes in a patient's overall functioning. How is your patient presenting during their visit? Are they reporting missing work or school or that they have stopped going to classes or other usual social activities? This is when we want you to pay more attention to these symptoms, move into our assessment to identify the level of risk and safety plan, and identify additional supportive resources for the patient. This is often a challenging and intimidating area for many healthcare and medical providers to assess [2].

If you are concerned about a patient being at risk for suicide, some red flags or direct verbal cues may include statements like this:

J. Rose-Smith et al., *The Psychosocial Impact of Rheumatic Conditions*, https://doi.org/10.1007/978-3-031-95338-5_3

- "I want to go to sleep and never wake up."
- "I am better off dead."
- "My family will be better without me."
- "No one will notice that I am even gone, I am so alone."

It is important to further assess statements or warning signs shared by patients, by exploring further what the patient means. Some possible questions to ask include the following:

- What do you mean by not wanting to wake up?
- Can you tell me more?
- Have you felt this way before?
- I'm concerned/worried. Can I ask you a few more questions?

Talking about these feelings will not put the idea of suicide in someone's head. If they are thinking of hurting themselves, they are already thinking about it. If they have had those ideas, they have had them before this conversation. Asking these challenging questions gives you a chance to understand and assess their level of risk. It also allows patients to give voice to their feelings and ideas.

Many studies show that people have ambivalence about committing suicide [3]. You cannot make or ultimately stop someone from hurting themselves, but there is a definite probability of preventing someone from doing so by asking the questions, assessing their immediate danger, and understanding if these feelings are passive or part of their depression. Remember you are part of a team, and seeking support from your interdisciplinary colleagues is necessary to help you assess and intervene with patients identifying with suicide risk.

Mental Health Screeners

A mental health screening is a set of questions that are provided to patients to support healthcare and mental health providers screening for mental health conditions. The information gained from these tools help providers learn about a person's mood, thinking, and behavior. There are great tools to help screen and identify mental health conditions early. More recently, studies have highlighted the value of incorporating depression screenings at rheumatology visits. These screenings invite patients to talk about their mental health concerns and permit earlier detection of these concerns. "The simple act of offering depression screening at every visit has helped create a culture that 'normalizes' or almost 'de-stigmatizes' mental health issues by folding it into their routine visit" [4]. There are a number of tools and screeners available that can be used to adapt to your specific setting. Below are some examples of mental health screeners to support you in your practice [5].

Mental Health Screeners to Support You in Your Practice

- **Patient Health Questionnaires Depression scale: PHQ-8 and PHQ9** are multipurpose instruments used for screening, diagnosing and monitoring, and measuring the severity of depression. The PHQ-8 differs from the more commonly used PHQ-9 in that it excludes the final question addressing suicidal ideation [6, 7].
- **Columbia-Suicide Severity Rating Scale (C-SSRS):** a short questionnaire that can be administered quickly in the field by those with no formal mental health training, and it is relevant in a wide range of settings and for individuals of all ages. This scale has been translated into many languages and has been used in diverse settings ranging from hospitals, primary care offices, schools, and colleges [8, 9].
- **Beck Depression Inventory**: self-reported 21-item questionnaire used to measure the severity of depression. It has been modified, and there is a shortened version of this tool, the Beck Depression Inventory Fast Screen (BDI-FS), that can be used in different clinical settings [10, 11].

- **Hospital Anxiety and Depression Scale (HADS):** a self-assessment 14-item scale used to identify states of depression and anxiety in hospital settings and outpatient medical clinics. HADS targets nonphysical symptoms so that it can be used to diagnose depression in people with significant physical health concerns [12, 13].
- **PROMIS® (Patient Reported Outcomes Measurement Information System):** set of measures created by the National Institutes of Health that evaluates and monitors physical, mental, and social health in adults and children across health conditions. PROMIS has developed items banks that are relevant to rheumatology, can be modified to a patient or a practice, and are currently widely available[1] [14].

References

1. Gürhan N, Beşer NG, Polat Ü, Koç M. Suicide risk and depression in individuals with chronic illness. Community Ment Health J. 2019;55(5):840–8.
2. Oquendo MA, Bernanke JA. Suicide risk assessment: tools and challenges. World Psychiatry. 2017;16(1):28–9.
3. Heinsch M, Sampson D, Huens V, Handley T, Hanstock T, Harris K, et al. Understanding ambivalence in help-seeking for suicidal people with comorbid depression and alcohol misuse. PLoS One. 2020;15(4):e0231647.
4. Saltzman H. The power of asking: mental health screening in pediatric rheumatology us: rheumatology advisor. 2021. https://www.rheumatologyadvisor.com/home/topics/pediatric-rheumatology/mental-health-screening-pediatric-rheumatology-hanna-saltzman-carra/. Accessed 26 Apr 2023.
5. ElSherbiny DA, ElSayed SW. Depression in rheumatoid arthritis patients: screening for a frequent yet underestimated comorbidity. Egyp Rheumatol. 2020;42(2):89–93.
6. Shin C, Lee SH, Han KM, Yoon HK, Han C. Comparison of the usefulness of the PHQ-8 and PHQ-9 for screening for major depressive disorder: analysis of psychiatric outpatient data. Psychiatry Investig. 2019;16(4):300–5.

[1] https://www.healthmeasures.net/explore-measurement-systems/promis. Last visited: 04-26-2023

7. Questionnaire. The Patient Health Questionnaire (PHQ-9) – overview: Pfizer Inc. 2023. https://www.drugsandalcohol.ie/26814/1/Patient%20Health%20Questionnaire.pdf. Accessed 21 Apr 2023.
8. Columbia. A simple set of 6 questions to screen for suicide: Columbia University Department of Psychiatry. 2021. https://www.columbiapsychiatry.org/news/simple-set-6-questions-screen-suicide. Accessed 26 Apr 2023.
9. Bjureberg J, Dahlin M, Carlborg A, Edberg H, Haglund A, Runeson B. Columbia-suicide severity rating scale screen version: initial screening for suicide risk in a psychiatric emergency department. Psychol Med. 2021;52(16):1–9.
10. Beck AT, Steer RA, Brown GK. BDI–FastScreen for medical patients. APA PsycTests; 2000.
11. Smarr KL, Keefer AL. Measures of depression and depressive symptoms: Beck depression inventory-II (BDI-II), Center for Epidemiologic Studies Depression Scale (CES-D), geriatric depression scale (GDS), hospital anxiety and depression scale (HADS), and patient health Questionnaire-9 (PHQ-9). Arthritis Care Res. 2011;63(S11):S454–S66.
12. Stern AF. The hospital anxiety and depression scale. Occup Med. 2014;64(5):393–4.
13. Zigmond AS, Snaith RP. The hospital anxiety and depression scale. Acta Psychiatr Scand. 1983;67(6):361–70.
14. Khanna D, Krishnan E, Dewitt EM, Khanna PP, Spiegel B, Hays RD. The future of measuring patient-reported outcomes in rheumatology: patient-reported outcomes measurement information system (PROMIS). Arthritis Care Res (Hoboken). 2011;63(Suppl 11):S486–90.

4 The Patient-Provider Partnership: It's a Dance!

Reflection: Keith's Story

The doctor walked in, introduced himself, sat down on the stool at eye level with the patient, and said, "Let me tell you what I know about your case." He spent three minutes or so recapping the patient's diagnosis, treatment, recorded complaints, and concerns including his demographics such as occupation and religion. The patient eyes widened, hanging on to his every word. When the doctor finished, he said, "Now tell me what I need to know about you and what's important to you." The patient looked stunned, but delighted. Tears welled up in his eyes as he replied, " I just want to rebound the ball to my son on the court a few more times." The doctor replied, "That will be the goal we focus on." Although faced with the reality of an aggressive illness and mounting symptoms, that day Keith felt hope. He felt *seen*. He walked out of that appointment and said, "He gets it. I am not this darn disease—I am still me."

The patient-provider relationship is a dance of sorts; the partners must be in lockstep as they navigate the changes in the music, the tempo, and the beat, to create a pleasurable experience. Similarly, doctors and patients must be in lockstep as they navigate the changes in symptoms and diagnosis, while considering the risks and benefits of treatments—and balancing what's important to the patient in their lives, including their families/caregivers.

J. Rose-Smith et al., *The Psychosocial Impact of Rheumatic Conditions*, https://doi.org/10.1007/978-3-031-95338-5_4

Navigating this relationship successfully can optimize care and well-being. However, neglecting the importance of cultivating this relationship can lead to suboptimal patient outcomes.

Effective patient-provider communication is the hallmark of effective therapeutic relationships. Managing a rheumatic illness often comes with many layers of complication, uncertainty, anxiety, and fear; meanwhile, doctors and patients often must pivot from one treatment pathway to the next. Cultivating a therapeutic alliance grounded in empathy, optimal communication, and trust is necessary for success.

The goals of an effective patient-provider relationship include [1]:

- Information exchange about diagnosis, symptoms, patient history, values, and creating a treatment plan.
- Building trust.
- Ongoing education.
- Provide therapeutic instructions.
- Cultivating a partnership.

Research shows that a positive provider-patient relationship was correlated with higher patient satisfaction with treatment, feelings of illness being well managed and controlled, and more hopefulness and positive feelings about current health status and future health [2]. Studies done with rheumatology patients also demonstrated that patients who had better communication with their providers and participated more actively with their care providers had less cumulative organ damage due to SLE [3]. Other studies demonstrated that greater participation and optimal communication in the provider-patient relationship led to less nonadherence and fewer medication side effects, as well as better overall global health. Meanwhile, patients who did not have much trust in their physicians were more likely to have poorer health outcomes [1].

It's important to remember that communication is not only verbal but can be influenced by what both providers and patients bring to the table, such as healthcare beliefs, perceptions, attitudes, culture, and more. All these factors can influence the quality of the therapeutic relationship. Studies have shown that patients believed that their relationship with their doctors was important, desired to "be seen," wanted their perspective taken into consideration throughout the care process, needed to "be believed," wanted their lived experience of the illness to be considered, and sought to partner with a physician in creating the care plans [1]. Patients also valued trust as a currency for building strong therapeutic alliances, which included the availability of the provider, their demonstration of knowledge, coming to the right diagnosis, and providing valuable information throughout the diagnosis and treatment process [4].

However, often the patient perceives a significant difference in the power dynamic between patient and provider. This may lead to barriers to the patient-provider relationship. Patients are often not invited to be partners in care and receive diagnoses and treatment plans without their input being solicited or considered. Despite the evolution of medical care and the adoption of various technologies, optimal patient outcomes are still based on the quality of the one-on-one relationship between the provider and the patient. Like any successful relationship, that connection must be intentionally cultivated. Research shows that doctors frequently overestimate the quality of their communication with their patients over 50% of the time [5]. The patient-provider relationship is often likened to a dance because it takes two people to make it successful. Effective communication from either the patient or the doctor alone cannot achieve the goals of the therapeutic relationship; it must be a mutual, patient-centered, and provider-centered effort focused on achieving the intended goals [6].

Like many decisions in life, patients and providers must approach medical decision-making by weighing the cost and benefits. These costs can be financial, physical, or psychosocial. For example, a medication may offer a benefit in the form of reduced inflammation but also have a cost, such as an unwelcome side effect, such as nausea or loss of appetite. A key question in weighing costs and benefits is the value that the provider and patient each assign to these costs and benefits, which oftentimes are different [7]. If optimal communication is lacking, the answers to these questions are never answered or integrated into care planning. For example, many treatment regimens for lupus such as Plaquenil, methotrexate, steroids, CellCept, and Benlysta are all effective medications that, when well monitored, can manage lupus with good results, despite their potential side effects. When making medical decisions, doctors can use their years of experience to formulate an equation and weigh the costs and benefits of using a certain drug. However, a patient may read about the same drugs and their toxicity, have conversations with friends that had bad experiences or adverse reactions, and have questions about its impact on reproductive health, activities of daily living, or their ability to work. This can result in anxiety and fear leading to a decision to not take their treatment. The doctor should actively explore feelings and thoughts about treatments and invite conversations about the treatment plan to secure patient buy-in. These feelings can also be brought up with the doctor to enable an open discussion of the cost and benefits as perceived by the patient [7].

Patient-Provider Responsibilities

In the therapeutic alliance, both the provider and patient share responsibilities to help facilitate a harmonious dance.

Doctor's Responsibilities

- Keep doors of communication open to invite trust.
- Respect patients, their concerns, their time, and the pressures in their lives.
- Offer emotional support to patients.
- Be an advocate for your patient and be fully present.
- Recognize that, like every other relationship, care is a partnership.
- Educate patients about their illnesses and medications.
- Develop an office environment that is sensitive, supportive, caring, responsive, safe, and private (in compliance with the Health Insurance Portability and Accountability Act [HIPAA]).

- Keep up to date on medical knowledge and patient care.
- Review patient medications regularly.
- Minimize patient wait times.
- Establish a process for responding to problems, scheduling discussions, and arranging prescription refills. Emergencies should not be handled by email.
- Ensure that patients are satisfied with their care.
- Have knowledge of the current realities of the healthcare system, as well as policies that affect it, such as the Affordable Care Act. Know what this represents to the patient and to their specific illness and financial situation. Help the patient navigate through the complexities of the healthcare system. Appreciate medical costs and minimize them.
- Understand your patients and their lives.
- Return calls and other communications promptly.

Patient's Responsibilities

- Share your feelings honestly.
- Respect doctors, their concerns, their time, and the pressures in their lives. However, realize that you don't need to accept poor treatment.
- Let the doctor know who you are as a person.
- Help your doctor be your advocate.
- Accept your important role in the partnership.
- Have knowledge of your health condition and be an informed consumer of medical care.
- Maintain an up-to-date, detailed time chart, including all pertinent information regarding your healthcare, beginning with the last time you felt well and continuing up to the present day. This can be written by hand, typed into a computer file (such as a Microsoft Word or Excel document), or maintained using an app on your mobile phone or tablet.

- Know your medications, doses, reasons for taking them, and associated side effects. Be sure to tell your doctor which medications you are currently taking, including all prescriptions, over-the-counter medicines, health foods and supplements, or alternative medications.
- Tell your doctor which medications you have stopped. If you do not, the doctor may incorrectly believe that you have been taking it and that it is not working.
- Arrive on time and expect the same from your doctor.
- Report symptoms accurately and in a timely manner.
- Give feedback about your care. If you are unhappy with your care, say so!
- Communicate information about the costs of medicines and medical care.
- Be accurate and assertive with messages. You should specify the timeframe in which you need a response, as well as the type of response it should be (such as a phone call or email message) [7].

Disparities and Patient-Provider Communication

Disparities in how patients of color are treated relative to how White patients are treated within the context of doctor-patient visits are well documented. Disparities in patient-provider relationships can be fueled by bias and can result in mistrust, delays in healthcare access, decreased adherence to treatment plans, and patient dissatisfaction [8, 9]. In one study, communication disparities were present even after controlling for socioeconomic, health, and provider characteristics, demonstrating that providers were less likely to communicate information about incidental medical findings to patients of color relative to White patients [10].

Tools for Building Strong Patient-Provider Relationships

Given the numerous barriers to effective patient-provider communication—such as power imbalances, fear of challenging the expert provider, and factors like disparities, racism, and cultural norms—it's crucial to acknowledge these dynamics in order to foster a more therapeutic alliance. Integrating tools—such as those discussed below—that engage both patient and provider in the care process should be a key component of care delivery.

Studies suggest that providing training in communication skills and patient engagement resulted in important improvements in the patient-provider alliance and enhanced care outcomes [5].

Interventions to address disparities and improve communication at the patient-provider level are needed.

Shared Decision-Making

Shared decision-making is a key component of patient-centered healthcare. It is a process in which clinicians and patients work together to make decisions and select tests, treatments, and care plans based on clinical evidence that balances risks and expected outcomes with patient preferences and values [11]. Sometimes this can feel challenging to incorporate into practice due to time pressures, knowledge of the patient, and other barriers; however, below are a few techniques to enhance the ability to incorporate these techniques.

The Agency for Healthcare Research and Quality (AHRQ) has published several tools to assist providers in incorporating shared decision-making to enhance communication and promote optimal patient outcomes.

AHRQ's SHARE Approach is a five-step process for shared decision-making that includes exploring and comparing the benefits, harms, and risks of each option through meaningful dialogue about what matters most to the patient [12] (Fig. 4.1).

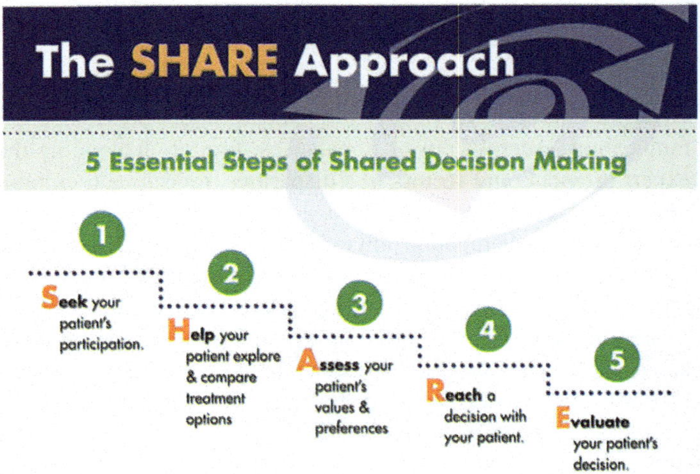

Fig. 4.1 The SHARE approach

Preparing Patients to Be Engaged in Care

Research shows that when patients wrote down an agenda before their primary care visit, 74% of clinicians and 79% of patients agreed that communication during the visit improved. More than 80% of the clinicians in the study wanted patients to continue to write down an agenda. The "Be Prepared. Be Engaged" strategy encourages patients and their families to prepare for and become more fully engaged in their medical appointments. The goal is to help patients and families set their visit agenda and to *be ready*, *speak up*, and *ask questions* [13] (Figs. 4.2 and 4.3).

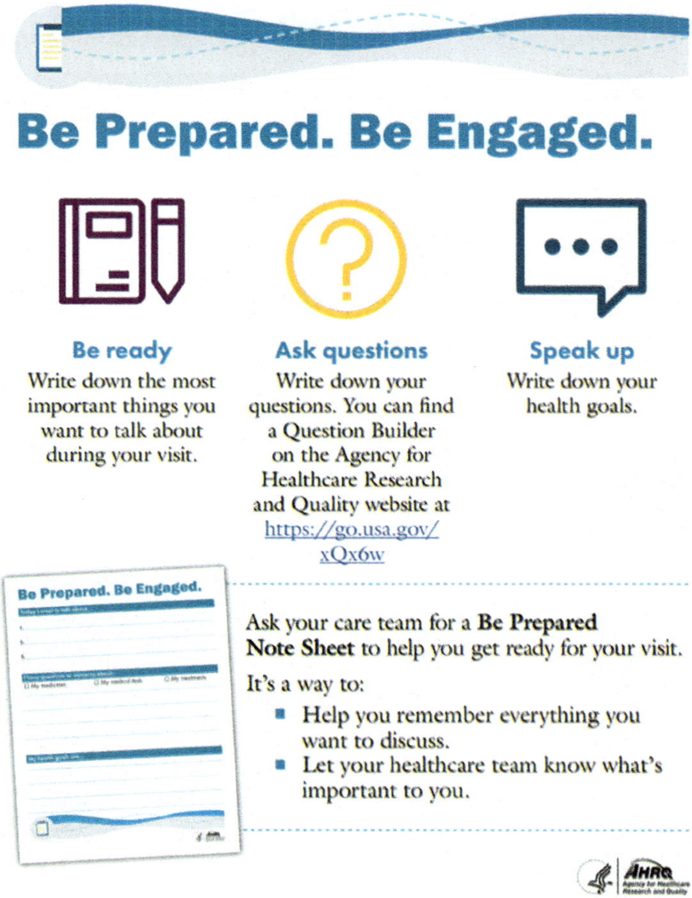

Fig. 4.2 Be Prepared patient flyer [14]

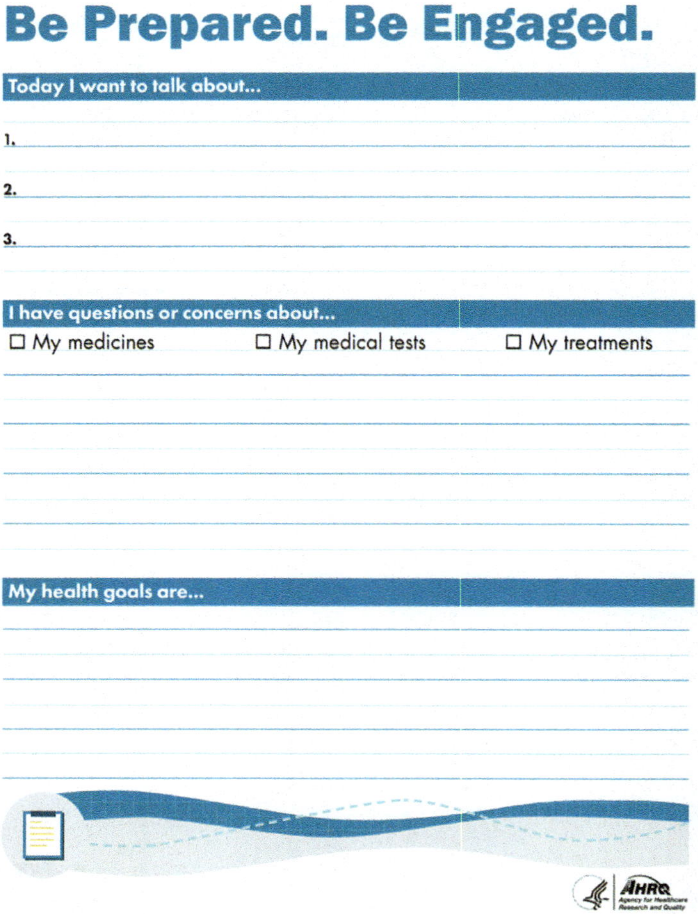

Be Prepared. Be Engaged.

Today I want to talk about...

1.
2.
3.

I have questions or concerns about...

☐ My medicines ☐ My medical tests ☐ My treatments

My health goals are...

AHRQ
Agency for Healthcare Research and Quality

Fig. 4.3 Be Prepared note sheet [14]

Motivational Interviewing

Motivational interviewing is a person-centered conversation style used to engage patients in behavior change by learning about their ambivalence and resistance and strengthening their own motivation to change. The four key motivational interviewing techniques that are demonstrated below can help providers achieve enhanced patient engagement and help move patients toward important decision-making and actual change [15].

Case Example: Using Open-Ended Questions, Affirmation, Reflective Listening, and Summarization (OARS)

A patient with lupus is hesitant to start Plaquenil despite ongoing recommendations by her rheumatologist. Patient reports that she is "afraid of being on medication forever."

- **Open-Ended Questions**
  Provider: "I'm following up with you because your rheumatologist shared with me that you have questions about Plaquenil."
  Patient: "Yes, I don't want to take that medicine."
  Provider: "What are some of your concerns?"
  Patient: "I've heard it can mess with your eyes. I'm scared about that. I have talked to my doctor about it."
- **Affirmation:**
  Provider: "It's reasonable for you to feel scared and it's difficult to try something new.
  Patient: "Yes, I know, but I still worry about the side effects even though I know it will help my lupus."
- **Reflective Listening:**
  Provider: "It's helpful that you were able to tell your doctor about your concerns and I'm wondering if it's possible to think about what may help you feel more comfortable starting this medicine."

Patient: "I would feel better if my doctor would tell me what my chances are of my eyes being affected. Even then, I still don't want to be on medication forever."

- **Summarization:**

Provider: "We just talked about some of your worries about starting Plaquenil and that you would feel better having another conversation with your doctor about it. Would you be able to do so?"

Teach-Back Method

When managing a rheumatic illness, we are often asking patients to take in and understand a large amount of complex medical information as they work toward making decisions about treatment and various medical interventions. This can often lead to confusion and distress. The teach-back method focuses on asking patients to share with the provider in their own words what the provider told them. The teach-back method is used to verify patient's understanding of the health information they are provided. It involves asking patients to explain in their own words what a health provider has just told them. This technique has been proven to improve patient satisfaction, knowledge, skills, and self-care abilities in patients with chronic disease [16]. Research shows that teach-back was found to be effective across a wide range of settings, populations, and outcome measures [16].

Addressing health literacy is also a key component to building viable patient-provider relationships. Research shows that around 35% of Americans had lower than an intermediate level of health literacy [17]. Low health literacy is connected to increased health system use and costs, health disparities, and poor health outcomes, especially for patients with chronic illnesses managing complex healthcare plans [17]. The Agency for Healthcare Research and Quality (AHRQ) also endorses teach-back as a safety strategy and a strategy for addressing health literacy.

Try the Teach-Back Method

- **Keep in mind this is not a test of the patient's knowledge**. It is a test of how well you explained the information or concept.
- **Plan your approach**. Think about how you will ask your patients to teach-back the information. For example:
  - "We covered a lot today and I want to make sure that I explained things clearly. So, let's review what we discussed. Can you please describe the 3 things you agreed to do to help you control your diabetes?"
- "**Chunk and Check**." Don't wait until the end of the visit to initiate teach-back. Chunk out information into small segments and have your patient teach it back. Repeat several times during a visit.
- **Clarify and check again**. If teach-back uncovers a misunderstanding, explain things again using a different approach. Ask patients to teach-back again until they are able to correctly describe the information in their own words. If they parrot your words back to you, they may not have understood.
- **Start slowly and use consistently**. At first, you may want to try teach-back with the last patient of the day. Once you are comfortable with the technique, use teach-back with everyone, every time!
- **Practice**. It will take a little time, but once it is part of your routine, teach-back can be done without awkwardness and does not lengthen a visit.
- **Use the show-me method**. When prescribing new medicines or changing a dose, research shows that even when patients correctly say when and how much medicine they'll take, many will make mistakes when asked to demonstrate the dose. You could say, for example:
  - "I've noticed that many people have trouble remembering how to take their blood thinner. Can you show me how you are going to take it?"

- **Use handouts along with teach-back**. Write down key information to help patients remember instructions at home. Point out important information by reviewing written materials to reinforce your patients' understanding. You can allow patients to refer to handouts when using teach-back, but make sure they use their own words and are not reading the material back verbatim [18].

References

1. Georgopoulou S, Prothero L, D'Cruz DP. Physician-patient communication in rheumatology: a systematic review. Rheumatol Int. 2018;38(5):763–75.
2. Beusterien K, Bell JA, Grinspan J, et al. Physician-patient interactions and outcomes in systemic lupus erythematosus (SLE): a conceptual model. Lupus. 2013;22(10):1038–45.
3. Ward MM, Sundaramurthy S, Lotstein D, Bush TM, Neuwelt CM, Street RL Jr. Participatory patient-physician communication and morbidity in patients with systemic lupus erythematosus. Arthritis Rheum. 2003;49(6):810–8.
4. Haugli L, Strand E, Finset A. How do patients with rheumatic disease experience their relationship with their doctors? A qualitative study of experiences of stress and support in the doctor-patient relationship. Patient Educ Couns. 2004;52(2):169–74.
5. Ha JF, Longnecker N. Doctor-patient communication: a review. Ochsner J. 2010;10(1):38–43.
6. AHA Data. AHA annual survey database™ the most credible and consistent data about the Nation's Hospitals [Internet]. AHA Data & Insights. 2021. https://www.ahadata.com/aha-annual-survey-database. Accessed 27 Apr 2021.
7. Paget SA. Doctor-patient communication: guidelines and best practices: hospital for special surgery. 2019. https://www.hss.edu/conditions_doctor-patient-communication.asp#:~:text=a%20good%20doctor%3F-,Dr.,his%20or%20her%20treatment%20recommendations. Accessed 27 Apr 2021.
8. Blair IV, Steiner JF, Fairclough DL, Hanratty R, Price DW, Hirsh HK, et al. Clinicians' implicit ethnic/racial bias and perceptions of care among black and Latino patients. Ann Fam Med. 2013;11(1):43–52.

9. Beyer KM, Young S, Bemanian A. Persistent racial disparities in breast cancer mortality between black and white women: what is the role for structural racism? Geospatial approaches to energy balance and breast. Cancer. 2019:361–78.
10. Schut RA. Racial disparities in provider-patient communication of incidental medical findings. Soc Sci Med. 2021;277:113901.
11. Deniz S, Akbolat M, Çimen M, Ünal Ö. The mediating role of shared decision-making in the effect of the patient-physician relationship on compliance with treatment. J Patient Exp. 2021;8:23743735211018066.
12. AHRQ. The SHARE approach: a model for shared decisionmaking – fact sheet us: agency for healthcare research and quality, Rockville, MD. 2020. https://www.ahrq.gov/health-literacy/professional-training/shared-decision/tools/factsheet.html. Accessed 27 Apr 2021.
13. AHRQ. Guide to improving patient safety in primary care settings by engaging patients and families: agency for healthcare research and quality, Rockville, MD. 2021. https://www.ahrq.gov/patient-safety/reports/engage.html. Accessed 27 Apr 2021.
14. AHRQ. Be prepared. Be engaged: agency for healthcare research and quality, Rockville, MD. 2023. https://www.ahrq.gov/sites/default/files/wysiwyg/professionals/quality-patient-safety/patient-family-engagement/pfeprimarycare/beprepared-patient-notesheet-final508.pdf. Accessed 27 Apr 2021.
15. Miller WR, Rollnick S. Motivational interviewing: helping people change. Guilford Press; 2012.
16. Talevski J, Wong Shee A, Rasmussen B, Kemp G, Beauchamp A. Teach-back: a systematic review of implementation and impacts. PLoS One. 2020;15(4):e0231350.
17. Yen PH, Leasure AR. Use and effectiveness of the teach-Back method in patient education and health outcomes. Fed Pract. 2019;36(6):284–9.
18. AHRQ. Use the teach-back method: tool #5: agency for healthcare research and quality, Rockville, MD. 2020. https://www.ahrq.gov/health-literacy/improve/precautions/tool5.html. Accessed 27 Apr 2021.

5 Cultural Considerations and Addressing Patient Values

Can You See Me Now?
A patient with lupus once shared that she would show up to her doctor's appointment dressed in what she described as her "royal African fabrics." She described receiving stares from the administrative staff and experiencing low engagement, minimal eye contact, and a lack of warm interpersonal connection from her doctor. She described their interaction as, "a sort of business transaction, where information exchange was abrupt and treatment plans were very circumscribed." Upon leaving her appointment, she observed the doctor being very "chatty" with a male patient dressed in a suit. The next appointment she decided to wear her work clothes which she described as "Wall Street professional." Upon arriving to her appointment at check-in, she received a few compliments from the check-in staff, and they even asked if she wanted some water.

However, after entering the appointment with her doctor, he took a long pause, looked at her and went on to carry on the appointment in his usual fashion. She said upon leaving he did say, "It was good to see you. Have a nice day." At her next visit, she planned to address her concerns with her doctor. She wore her usual "off day attire, my royal African fabrics" and was prepared to let the doctor know he was treating her differently and question his professional style. As she sat in the exam room preparing her talking points, the doctor came in with a "feathered

J. Rose-Smith et al., *The Psychosocial Impact of Rheumatic Conditions*, https://doi.org/10.1007/978-3-031-95338-5_5

headdress and a vibrant colorful scarf." They both looked at each other and had what she described as a "belly laugh—we both saw each other that day."

Culture

Patients come to healthcare with a set of diverse beliefs, values, customs, lived experiences, attitudes, and behaviors that inform their worldview of illness, health, and healthcare. However, too often, these factors are not asked about and are ignored in the care of patients. Conversely, oftentimes we expect providers to check these ingrained parts of their realities at the door while caring for patients at the expense of engaging in fully empathic and genuine relationships with patients, which can impede high-quality care [1].

The patient and provider are both fully human, and we must recognize and normalize that they both are coming in with a set of systems, shared beliefs, values, customs, behavior, and artifacts that they may often use to cope with their world/realities. These factors are defined as culture, often passed from one generation to the next through learning. Culture can be influenced by many things, including religion, race, ethnic background, language, country of origin, age, and even technology. Culture is the lens or framework in which we view the world; it is central to what we see, how we make sense of what we experience, and how we express ourselves [2, 3].

According to the National CLAS (Culturally and Linguistically Appropriate Services) standards, cultural competency is one of the cornerstones to providing effective, quality care to patients with diverse beliefs, values, attitudes, and behaviors.[1] This requires healthcare systems and practices to be able to personalize healthcare according to cultural and linguistic differences. It also requires understanding the impact that cultural differences can

[1]https://thinkculturalhealth.hhs.gov/clas. Last Visited: 04-20-2023

have on how we deliver healthcare [4]. It requires us to *see* our patients and allow ourselves to *be seen* by them.

The Impact of Culture

Culture can determine:

- What is "normal".
- Why an illness is happening at this time.
- The meaning of symptoms and how to treat them.
- Who makes decisions in the family.
- When to stop and start treatment.
- The use of traditional/alternative medicines.
- The trustworthiness of a provider.
- How patients communicate.
- The uptake of technology.

Failure to address cultural issues can lead to:

- Feelings of not being seen or heard.
- Feeling isolated.
- Anxiety and worry.
- Poor patient-provider communication.
- Nonadherence.
- Helplessness.
- Loss to follow-up.
- Poor patient outcomes.

These factors should be considered, especially when caring for patients with rheumatic illness, whose journey to care is often fraught with misdiagnoses, failed treatments, and lack of specialty providers. Additionally, they frequently struggle to manage symptoms that are overlooked or dismissed due to the complexities of conditions like lupus. In the face of uncertainty and no clear answers, patients have reported leaning into traditional practices and beliefs to make sense of their experiences and trying alternative pathways for treatment and symptom relief in an attempt to gain control of their symptoms and fight the betrayal they feel in their bodies.

> I tried everything—pills, potions, prayers, acupuncture, witchcraft … I just wanted to feel in control again. I was in so much pain my desperation led to seeking anything from those who listened to me.
> –Patient with RA and lupus

How Do We Get There? Ask and Share

Ask! It's important that we are curious about who our patients are and what they bring into healthcare. Not understanding how cultural practices and health beliefs can influence the way that care is perceived and received can often lead to poor outcomes. Asking about religion, cultures, and customs and doing some appropriate sharing affirm the patient's existence, experiences, and values. Equally important is clinicians bringing their own humanity and values into the room, which can be a conduit to building trust and mutual respect. These are all invaluable tools for engaging patients in a partnership so that, together, you can devise treatment plans that align with the patient's values and the provider's expertise, garnering their investment and follow-through.

Tips for Asking About Culture and Values

Asking patients about their health and cultural beliefs is a tool to help inform medical decision-making and permit seeing the patient as a whole person. Be sure to include these questions in formal medical assessments and document patient responses in the medical record. For example:

- "Is there anything I should know about your culture, beliefs, or religious practices that would help me take better care of you?"
- "What do you think caused your illness and how do you describe your experience with these symptoms? Do other

people in your family think it's caused by something else or call it something different?"
- "To help create the best nutrition plan for you, can you share with me what you usually cook at home?"
- "Do you have any dietary restrictions that we should consider as we develop a food plan to help you lose weight?"
- "Outside of prescription medications and over-the-counter treatments, what else do you use to treat your illness?"
- "Is there anyone else you would like to be here with you? Is there anyone I should talk with who helps you make medical decisions?"
- "Do you work with any holistic medicine doctors or traditional healers to advise you about your health?" [5].

Be Aware/Keep in Mind

These questions are not meant to "put patients into a box" or create stereotypes. Instead, they are meant to expand the provider's view of the patient's world and foster understanding of what is valuable to them. By asking these questions, providers can foster better patient engagement and incorporate cultural values and beliefs into the development of appropriate treatment plans. This approach facilitates mutual investment and ensures the plan reflects the patient in the context of their own realities and values. Asking these questions can provide invaluable information that helps providers personalize care to achieve the highest quality and most optimal outcomes [5].

Cultural Humility: A Journey

In a world where connectivity to global populations is easier and faster than ever, achieving cultural competence is more daunting than ever before. As providers, it is not realistic to know everything about every culture. However, making a commitment to cultural humility is more achievable and beneficial to caring for patients. Cultural humility is described as "entering a relationship with another person with the intention of honoring their beliefs, customs, and values" [6]. Most of us have heard the saying, "Treat others as you would like to be treated." Cultural humility, instead, encourages us to treat others the way *they* would like to be treated. This stance encourages us to engage in a process of self-exploration that necessitates examining our own values and beliefs and even challenging the beliefs we hold. It also demands a willingness to take a stance of curiosity with our patients, exercising a desire to learn from them and get to know who they are with the goal of providing the best care.

Cultural knowledge is the start of the journey in optimizing care with patients; cultivating an interpersonal relationship with patients by first understanding what we bring to the table as providers is essential. Engaging in self-evaluation and then moving to a place of curiosity to learn who our patients are and work to create an environment of respect, sensitivity, and openness can help to address complex issues that often come up in diverse relationships. Some of these issues include the patient-provider power imbalance, poor communication, lack of understanding, and lack of buy-in in the treatment plan which is critical for success.

The key question we must ask as we seek to practice from a place of cultural humility is: "What is important to the patient?" This question allows providers to bring the patient squarely into the room and at the center of their care. Oftentimes the provider knows the best treatment pathway and evidence-based clinical interventions that would optimize a patient's health outcomes. However, with no buy-in from the patient, that plan can fail. Research shows that most treatment plans fail due to poor communication, lack of relationship between doctor and patient, and barriers to cultural and language norms [7]. As quoted by W. J. Mayo: "The best interest of the patient is the only interest to be considered, and in order that the sick may have the benefit of advancing knowledge, union of forces is necessary" [8]. Joining forces with patients by cultivating knowledge, fostering curiosity, and inviting them to be valuable partners in care allows us to create mutually respectful and trusting relationships that lead to better patient outcomes.

Assessing What's Important to the Patient

- Set clear expectations that care will be a collaborative process.
  - Reassure the patient through words and actions that you are committed to understanding their needs and co-creating a tailored treatment plan. Emphasize that this is a collaborative process requiring their input, facilitated by open communication.
- Ask for the patient's input on collaborating in healthcare decisions.
  - Encourage decision-making, even small ones, to reinforce that you value their preferences, and help them feel comfortable expressing healthcare needs.
- Ask the patient about their goals to guide the treatment plan.
  - Model creation of the treatment plan by asking the patient about what they would to like to accomplish, and help them consider possible methods for achieving these goals.
- Use a strengths-based perspective.
  - Identify strengths, interests, and resilience factors that can be used to help the patient make difficult decisions and encourage engagement in the treatment plan.
- Ask the patient what they feel would be helpful in their care.
  - Inquire about any cultural practices or herbal remedies they've tried—what were the results? Are there religious, cultural, or individual convictions that influence their treatment choices?
- During the session, check if the patient needs clarification on any information they feel the provider didn't appropriately explain, or they didn't fully understand.
  - If using an interpreter, ensure they are interpreting the full discussion, not summarizing, as this can lose important nuance and meaning.
- After the session, ask the patient if they felt understood, if they followed the process, and if there is anything else they would like to add to be better understood.

- Clarify the patient's preferences regarding family involvement, and, depending on the patient's age, ability, and literacy, determine what information will be communicated to the family [6].

Implicit Bias

Two landmark reports by the Institute of Medicine, *Crossing the Quality Chasm* (2001) and *Unequal Treatment* (2002), highlighted pervasive racial and ethnic disparities in the US healthcare system [9, 10]. The reports found that even when patients had the same insurance and socioeconomic status as nonminorities—and when comorbidities, stage of presentation, and other confounders were controlled for—minorities often received lower-quality healthcare. Research shows that part of what causes disparities are the implicit biases of healthcare workers, which can unintentionally lead to providing lower-quality care for patients. Implicit biases are unconscious and can affect all of us and can have many consequences, including facilitating barriers to patient-provider relationships and impacting clinical care outcomes [11]. It's important that providers learn more about implicit bias, examine their own biases, and work to debias their interactions and interventions to optimize patient care and address known disparities that especially plague diverse and under-resourced patients.

In Summary

At the center of becoming a more culturally competent provider is our ability to "see" our patients. To do this, providers must invest in a journey of cultural humility, address their own biases, use a bio-psycho-social approach to help put patients at the center of care, see them as unique individuals and not stereotypes, and maintain respectful relationships that are built on our exploration of our patients' values, beliefs, and understanding of illness. This allows providers to foster more inclusive and equitable relationships with patients. Although this is not a complete solution to address disparities in care and inequalities, it serves as a key step toward reducing bias. By valuing patient input and understanding what matters most to them, we can foster better communication and trust—ultimately leading to improved care outcomes.

References

1. Trust HRE. Becoming a culturally competent health care organization: health research & educational trust; 2013. Available from: http://www.hpoe.org/Reports-HPOE/becoming_culturally_competent_health_care_organization.PDF. Accessed 20 Apr 2023.
2. Swihart DL, Yarrarapu SNS, Martin RL. Cultural religious competence in clinical practice. StatPearls. Treasure Island (FL): StatPearls Publishing Copyright © 2023, StatPearls Publishing LLC; 2023.
3. Swihart DL, Yarrarapu SNS, Martin RL. Cultural religious competence in clinical practice. 2018.
4. Brach C, Hall K, Fitall E. Cultural competence and patient safety. 2019. https://psnet.ahrq.gov/perspective/cultural-competence-and-patient-safety. Accessed 20 Apr 2023.
5. Rockville M. Consider culture, customs, and beliefs: tool #10. 2020. https://www.ahrq.gov/health-literacy/improve/precautions/tool10.html. Accessed 20 Apr 2023.
6. Stubbe DE. Practicing cultural competence and cultural humility in the care of diverse patients. Focus. 2020;18(1):49–51.
7. Toole J, Kohansieh M, Khan U, Romero S, Ghali M, Zeltser R, et al. Does your patient understand their treatment plan? Factors affecting patient understanding of their medical care treatment plan in the inpatient setting. J Patient Exp. 2020;7(6):1151–7.
8. Mayo, W. J. The necessity of cooperation in medicine: an address delivered at the Rush Medical College commencement [press release]. Mayo Clinic: Saint Marys Hospital, 1910.
9. Institute of Medicine Committee on Quality of Health Care in America. Crossing the quality chasm: a new health system for the 21st century. Washington: National Academies Press; 2001.
10. Smedley BD, Stith AY, Nelson AR. Institute of Medicine Committee on U, Eliminating R, Ethnic Disparities in Health C. In: Unequal treatment: confronting racial and ethnic disparities in health care. Washington: National Academies Press; 2003.
11. Heath S. What is implicit bias, how does it affect healthcare? Patient engagement hit. 2020.

Special Populations in Rheumatology: LGBTQIA+ Identity

6

Patient Stories

Andy, a Pediatric Patient

A 16-year-old patient with lupus comes in for their first appointment to see Dr. Y, a pediatric rheumatologist, for a consultation. They are accompanied to their appointment by their grandmother. Dr. Y asks their grandmother to step out of the room—as they do with all adolescent patients—so she can ask some questions to X in private. "Can you actually call me 'Andy?' That's what all my friends call me at school. I told Gram but she hates it- she says I'm just a tomboy because I have all brothers, so she still calls me 'Ashley.'"

Frank, an Adult Patient

Frank, who comes to the hospital frequently for treatment of his RA, has been misgendered multiple times when he checks in for his appointments by staff who use the pronouns "she" and "miss/ma'am." During his recent admitting process for surgery, the patient overheard staff referring to him as "she" multiple times. Frank felt disheartened that staff didn't get this right as this has happened to him many times before at other healthcare institu-

J. Rose-Smith et al., *The Psychosocial Impact of Rheumatic Conditions*, https://doi.org/10.1007/978-3-031-95338-5_6

tions. Feeling very upset, the patient told the staff member that his correct pronouns are "he/him/his," and that staff are not using the right pronouns. The staff member apologized and noted that this information was incorrect in the system. The staff member proceeded to review the information with the patient in the electronic health record to make sure this information was corrected.

Both Andy and Frank's cases are just two examples of the kinds of experiences that can be faced by patients who identify on the lesbian, gay, bisexual, transgender, queer/questioning, intersex, asexual, or other sex/gender minorities (LGBTQIA+) spectrum. In both of these cases, the patients went by different names or pronouns and indicated how they would like to be addressed to members of their healthcare team. In Andy's case, their rheumatologist created the space for Andy to disclose this information in private, despite his grandmother not being supportive of their identity. In Frank's case, he was repeatedly misgendered by staff due to how he presented, even though he has been seen frequently by the hospital. Despite the organization also having the ability to capture this information, the patient's pronouns were missed, which points to the fact that systems are not foolproof. These incidents negatively impacted his overall experience and engagement in care. As rheumatology professionals, we have a responsibility to be attuned to these issues to ensure we are providing holistic and affirming care to diverse populations.

Background

According to federal law, discrimination due to one's gender identity or sexual orientation is prohibited. Section 1557 of the Affordable Care Act explicitly prohibits discrimination based on "race, color, national origin, age, disability, or sex (including pregnancy, sexual orientation, gender identity, and sex characteristics), in covered health programs or activities" [1, 2]. This regulation was challenged in 2020 by the Trump administration's final rule, which "deleted the 2016 ACA rule definition of sex discrimination that included gender identity and sex stereotyping" [3]; however, soon after US Supreme Court issued a landmark ruling in *Bostock v. Clayton County, Georgia* [4]. It held that Title VII of the Civil Rights Act of 1964's prohibition on employment discrimination on the basis of sex includes discrimination based on sexual orientation and gender identity (SOGI) [5].

Within the past two decades, healthcare institutions and governing bodies have recognized disparities within the LGBTQIA+ population and have called healthcare organizations to assess and address the needs of LGBTQIA+ patients. In 2011 The Joint Commission released a field guide for US hospitals—*Advancing Effective Communication Cultural Competence and Patient- and Family-Centered Care: For the Lesbian, Gay, bisexual and Transgender (LGBT) Community*—which provided strategies, recommendations, and resources for the provision of patient-centered care for LGBT patients [6]. Additionally, the Institute of Medicine, now the National Academy of Medicine, published a report on the state of LGBTQ healthcare in the United States, which also identified the need to expand sex and gender minority health research [7]. Addressing LGBT health was also a priority area for Healthy People 2020 and continues to be a goal for Healthy People 2030 to "improve the health, safety, and well-being of lesbian, gay, bisexual and transgender (LGBT) individuals" [8].

Research shows that people who identify as LGBTQIA+ face several documented health-related challenges and disparities, including higher rates of physical and mental health problems, including depression, suicidality, substance use, and higher rates of cardiovascular disease. Disparities are even deeper for those in the transgender community, who experience higher rates of stigma, discrimination, and violence [9]. According to the 2015 Transgender Survey, 23% reported that they avoided seeking healthcare due to fear of discrimination and mistreatment by healthcare providers, with transgender people of color reporting higher rates of avoidance [10]. In the National Transgender Discrimination Survey (2011), the report found that nearly 20 percent of respondents had been refused medical care, one-third reported being discriminated against during a medical encounter, and 50 percent had to teach their medical providers about transgender care. More than 40 percent of participants have or will attempt suicide in their lifetime. Furthermore, about one in three transgender and gender-nonconforming Americans have experienced homelessness in their lifetimes [11].

These disparities, coupled with nondiscrimination laws and a call to action from leading healthcare institutions, support the need to provide affirming, inclusive, and safe care to LGBTQIA+ patients, who have a higher risk of certain health conditions, lack of access to care and negative experiences in healthcare environments.

LGBTQIA+ Identity and Rheumatology

Rheumatology professionals may ask: why does this matter? Is this significant in my area of specialty? The answer to this is yes—your knowledge and awareness of LGBTQIA+ health issues and your engagement with the patient in understanding their identity can significantly impact patient care.

Reproductive health, where one's gender identity and sexual orientation can be discussed, is a relevant topic for patients with rheumatic conditions, especially in pediatric rheumatology, where adolescent and young adult patients have identified topics such as "medication safety, sexual activity, family planning, peer relations and dating" [12] as important. Rheumatic disease patients often see their rheumatologists more frequently than their primary care provider (PCP), especially when treating active disease, and they develop longstanding relationships with their rheumatologists. This trusted patient-provider partnership can create the ideal opportunity to discuss these sensitive topics.

According to pediatric rheumatology experts, questions such as gender identity and sexual orientation can be asked within the context of the HEADSSS Assessment, which is a review of systems for adolescents which covers home environment, education, and sexuality, to name a few [12, 13]. Knowing this information and being sensitive to how a patient identifies can help the rheumatology care team to provide tailored treatment to the patient.

Additionally, there are health implications related to reproductive health and medications that one may be taking to affirm one's gender. It's important to understand if a patient who had a female sex assigned at birth but now identifies as a man, for example, still has a viable uterus and plans to become pregnant since certain medications such as methotrexate are teratogenic and unsafe for pregnancy. Additionally, there are some concerns in rheumatology around the use of gender-affirming hormone therapy impacting disease activity, although more research needs to be done in this space [14]. It's important that hormone treatments are managed appropriately by a physician to minimize health risks.

Terms to Know

There are several terms used by the LGBTQIA+ community that are important to be familiar with in order to provide the highest quality and affirming care to LGBTQIA+ patients. It's key to remember that terms change over time. Terms that are embraced today were not always welcomed by the community in the past, and terms that were more widely used a few years ago are now considered outdated. Below are a few terms to know, adapted from the National LGBTQIA+ Health Education Center [15]:

- *Chosen Name/Name Used:* The name a person goes by and wants others to use in personal communication, even if it is different from the name on that person's insurance or identification documents (e.g., birth certificate, driver's license, and passport).
- *Pronouns:* Pronouns are the words people should use when they are referring to you but not using your name.
- *Gender Identity:* A person's inner sense of being a girl/woman/female, boy/man/male, something else, or having no gender.
- *Sex Assigned at Birth:* The sex (male or female) assigned to an infant, most often based on the infant's anatomical and other biological characteristics. Sometimes referred to as birth sex, natal sex, biological sex, or sex; however, sex assigned at birth is the recommended term.
- *Transgender:* Describes a person whose gender identity and sex assigned at birth do not correspond based on traditional expectations. Transgender can also include people with gender

identities outside the girl/woman and boy/man gender binary structure, for example, people who are gender fluid or nonbinary. Sometimes abbreviated as trans.
- *Gender Diverse:* Describes the community of people who fall outside of the gender binary structure (e.g., nonbinary, genderqueer, gender fluid people).
- *Gender Expression:* The way a person communicates their gender to the world through mannerisms, clothing, speech, behavior, etc. Gender expression varies depending on culture, context, and historical period.
- *Sexual Orientation:* How a person characterizes their emotional and sexual attraction to others.

Direct Practice

Critical to caring for patients with rheumatology conditions is to understand the intersections of identities that one holds. A patient's identity as gay, lesbian, trans, etc., is only one of several identities a person has, and as healthcare providers, it's important that we recognize the intersection of these identities, which can impact how patients experience healthcare and understand one's illness. One must start from a stance of self-awareness, openness, dignity, and respect.

Recognize Your Privilege As a provider in the patient-provider relationship, one must recognize the power imbalance that exists between you and the patients you serve. You hold an inherent privilege of treating (or withholding treatment from) patients who rely on your expert knowledge and guidance to improve and enhance their well-being.

Be Aware of Your Own Biases Everyone has their own biases, whether explicit or implicit, and these biases—intentional or not—can impact your care for patients. Before even jumping into the "to dos" when caring for LGBTQIA+ patients, you must make a commitment to do the internal work of reflecting, examining, and identifying your own biases in order to begin to address them. Please see Chap. 5 for more information about the tools and resources you can use to address implicit biases.

Don't Make Assumptions Have you ever received an email from someone and been unsure of their title, such as whether they are a Miss, Mister, or something else, based on just their name or email address? This especially matters when serving the LGBTQIA+ community. As a society, we have been socialized to make automatic judgments (implicit bias) about whether one is male or female based on how we perceive them. We'll determine how to address them instead of *asking them* how they want to be addressed. The same goes for one's family members or romantic partnerships and making heteronormative assumptions—for example, assuming a male would be accompanied by his wife or that a child would have a mother and a father. Instead of making assumptions and risk making a mistake, we should simply ask. Misgendering a patient or making incorrect assumptions about who they brought to an appointment, for example, is harmful, especially when the same mistakes are made repeatedly by multiple providers in their life.

Use Gender-Neutral Language We are often socialized to ask questions that are rooted in heteronormativity and cisnormativity. Building on best practices to avoid making assumptions, when one asks questions related to one's gender identity, their support system, or their romantic partnerships, it's best to use gender-neutral language. Some examples follow: (a) You notice your male patient brought a male-presenting person with them to his appointment. You can simply ask: "Who did you bring with you to your appointment today?" to let the patient tell you who they are. (b) Instead of saying "mother" or "father," you can say "parent or guardian." (c) Instead of saying, "do you have a boyfriend/girlfriend/husband/wife?" you can say, "do you have a partner/spouse?"

Follow the Patient's Lead As previously mentioned, patients who go to you for care have different experiences and identities, and it's important that one does not treat a patient who identifies as LGBTQIA+ differently than those who do not identify with the community. You should explore a patient's gender identity and sexual orientation as it relates to their presenting health issue. A nonbinary patient may not want to explore this every time they come for a visit, and to do so would be inappropriate and could be interpreted as unnecessarily intrusive. It's important to respect boundaries set by the patient in order to provide the most affirming care possible.

Use the Language Your Patients Use Be attentive to how your patient describes themselves and their body parts. Use the language they use to describe different parts of their body. For example, a transgender male patient may describe their breasts as "chest," and as their provider, you should use this same language.

Use a Trauma-Informed Approach Given that people who identify as LGBTQIA+ experience higher risks of trauma, as described previously, a trauma-informed approach can enhance the care provided to this community, lead to a more accurate understanding of the clinical case, and determine the appropriate treatment. According to Substance Abuse and Mental Health Services (SAMHSA), the principles of trauma-informed care include safety, trustworthiness and transparency, peer support, collaboration and mutuality, empowerment, voice and choice, and cultural, historical, and gender issues [16].

Consider the Patient's Support System As with any patient, with the patient's permission, one's family and support system should be included in care. As mentioned, many LGBTQIA+ individuals face discrimination or bias in healthcare, and one way this can show up for LGBTQIA+ patients is when they have a partner of the same gender. A provider may make an incorrect assumption that the patient's partner or spouse is a "friend" or not recognize the patient's partner as a caregiver. The inclusion of the patient's same-sex spouse can improve health outcomes and disease management so they are better prepared to support the patient [17].

Continue Learning Regardless of how many LGBTQIA+ patients you see or don't see, it's important to continue learning about LGBTQIA+ health concerns—especially in rheumatology, relevant terminology, and best practices in caring for LGBTQIA+ patients. Because of the stigma the community faces and a history of negative experiences in healthcare, more people likely identify as LGBTQIA+ than are reported at your organization. Some patients may not be out to their provider due to fear of mistreatment. It's therefore critical to be prepared to serve those who identify with the community and to create safe spaces for patients to bring their whole selves to their care. You never know who is going to walk through your door!

Organizational and Macro-Level Interventions

In order to best care for and advocate for rheumatology patients who identify as LGBTQIA+, we must ensure that we are addressing LGBTQIA+ health on an organizational/institutional level by implementing policies, guidelines, and practices that support LGBTQIA+ patients and their families. The following are some macro-level strategies your organization or practice can take to foster an LGBTQIA+ inclusive environment.

Create Affirming Spaces Look around your practice, clinical exam rooms, the registration area, and the lobby. Is there anything that supports the LGBTQIA+ community? By adopting LGBTQIA+ pride flags, stickers, or imagery and posting them in public areas, you're communicating to patients that *you are welcome here*. One can use images for same-gender couples or nonbinary people so patients can see themselves reflected in your organization's brochures, commercials, and other marketing materials.

Form/Join a LGBTQIA+ Hospital-Wide Committee This committee, made up of stakeholders from across departments with a vested interest in enhancing care for LGBTQIA+ patients, can help monitor external trends related to LGBTQIA+ health and work to adopt practices to address LGBTQIA+ health equity. As part of one's diversity, equity, and inclusion strategy, one's organization can commit to applying for the Healthcare Equality Index (HEI), which is a "national LGBTQ+ benchmarking tool that evaluates healthcare facilities' policies and practices related to the equity and inclusion of their LGBTQ+ patients, visitors, and employees" [18]. Healthcare organizations that meet the requirements can achieve the Leader in LGBTQ+ Healthcare Equality designation, which can communicate to the public that the organization is LGBTQIA+ inclusive.

Implement Staff Trainings Staff training is critical in order to best serve LGBTQIA+ patients. Training must be mandatory, given regularly, and be provided to all staff, clinical and nonclinical, in order for the organization to see lasting change. Often this must be accompanied by a culture shift, driven by leadership and the external environment to drive an organization to focus on providing inclusive, affirming, and safe care to this patient population. Training should include why LGBTQIA+ inclusive and affirming healthcare is important, laws and regulations, how it aligns with the organization's mission and values, LGBTQIA+ health disparities, important terminology, how to engage with patients, use of inclusive and gender-neutral language, scripting language, and privacy/confidentiality issues. Organizations, such as the National LGBTQIA+ Health Education Center,[1] have a host of resources and publications to educate healthcare providers, allied health professionals, and administrative staff.

Collect Sexual Orientation and Gender Identity (SOGI) Data In order to identify the LGBTQIA+ health needs and health disparities faced at your healthcare institution, you must collect SOGI data to be able to invite LGBTQIA+ patients to self-identify. SOGI data includes a two-part question: gender identity and sex assigned at birth in addition to legal/administrative sex and sexual orientation. Typically, this information is part of the demographics

[1] https://www.lgbtqiahealtheducation.org/. Last visited: 04-26-2023.

section of one's medical record. It is important for SOGI data fields to continue to be a part of Certified Electronic Health Record Technology (CEHRT) products, according to the Office of the National Coordinator (ONC) for Health Information Technology [19]. Implementing SOGI data collection is a process that requires buy-in from your organization's leadership, collaboration with IT, and thorough education and training of staff. The National LGBTQIA+ Health Education Center has several resources to support this effort, including a guide for planning and implementation and educational information for staff and patients [20]. This data can be used to explore existing disparities as it relates to the provision of care and healthcare outcomes. An organization can stratify screenings, procedures, and outcomes by SOGI information to explore whether there are any differences in care provided to lesbian, gay, bisexual, or transgender patients versus non-LGBTQIA+ counterparts.

Create LGBTQIA+ Inclusive Policies Policies to support LGBTQIA+ patients and employees are critical to creating an inclusive environment. Some examples of key policies implemented include: [1] a rooming policy that requires patients to be roomed according to their gender identity and not their legal/administrative sex; [2] a policy to guide staff on asking about gender identity, sex assigned at birth, and sexual orientation questions to patients; [3] bathroom policy that explicitly allows patients to use the bathroom that aligns with their gender identity; and [4] employee insurance coverage that covers partners and gender-affirming care.

Enhance Your Systems (e.g., Electronic Health Records) to Be More Affirming Ensure that preferred/chosen names and pronouns are easily visible on your EHR so patients are addressed appropriately. By making this information more easily identifiable and integrating them into patient lists and hospital ID wristbands, patients are less likely to be misgendered. Staff training is critical here to educate staff about how to access this information, change it if needed, and utilize the information during patient interactions and when discussing patients. Additionally, systems can be set up to support the safety needs of patients who identify with a gender identity different from the sex assigned at birth. Best practice advisories to alert providers when this information does not match can help ensure that patients are offered clinically appropriate screening and counseling. For example, prior to surgery, a pregnancy test is given to all patients with a viable uterus regardless of their gender identity.

Obtain Feedback from the Community The needs of the LGBTQIA+ population in your community may be more specific or niche in your location. It's important to create patient advisory boards, review patient satisfaction and quality surveys regularly, and stratify feedback to see what organizations can do to better meet the needs of the LGBTQIA+ community in your area.

The above is a sampling of the many individual and macro-level strategies one can take to support LGBTQIA+ patients and their families in rheumatology. When we serve diverse populations of patients, it's important to invite patients to bring their multiple identities to their care, provide the space for one to self-identify, and recognize how these can shape one's experiences in healthcare and ultimately impact health outcomes.

References

1. US Department of Health and Human Services Section 1557 of the Patient Protection and Affordable Care Act Washington, DC: Government Printing Office: US Department of Health Human Services. 2016. https://www.hhs.gov/civil-rights/for-individuals/section-1557/index.html. Accessed 26 April 2023.
2. US Department of Health and Human Services. Summary: final rule implementing section 1557 of the affordable care act. Washington: US Department of Health and Human Services; 2016.
3. Cahill S, Miller AS, Keuroghlian AS. Sexual and gender minority health equity in the Biden administration. JAMA Health Forum. 2022;3(2):e214868.
4. Bostock v. Clayton County (2019).
5. US Department of Health and Human Services. Protecting the Rights of Lesbian, Gay, Bisexual, Transgender, Queer, and Intersex (LGBTQI+) People: Content created by Office for Civil Rights. 2023. https://www.hhs.gov/ocr/lgbtqi/index.html. Accessed 26 April 2023.

6. Guide AF. Advancing effective communication, cultural competence, and patient-and family-centered care for the lesbian, gay, bisexual, and transgender (LGBT) community: a field guide. Oak Brook: Joint Commission; 2011.
7. Garofalo R. The health of lesbian, gay, bisexual, and transgender people: building a foundation for better understanding. Washington: The National Academies Press; 2011.
8. US Department of Health and Human Services. Goal: Improve the health, safety, and well-being of lesbian, gay, bisexual, and transgender people: Health People 2023 coordinated by the Office of Disease Prevention and Health Promotion. 2023. https://health.gov/healthypeople/objectives-and-data/browse-objectives/lgbt. Accessed 26 Apr 2023.
9. Hughes TL, Jackman K, Dorsen C, Arslanian-Engoren C, Ghazal L, Christenberry-Deceased T, et al. How can the nursing profession help reduce sexual and gender minority related health disparities: recommendations from the National Nursing LGBTQ health summit. Nurs Outlook. 2022;70(3):513–24.
10. James S, Herman J, Rankin S, Keisling M, Mottet L, Anafi M. The report of the 2015 US transgender survey. Washington: NCTE. p. 2016.
11. Grant JM, Motter LA, Tanis J. Injustice at every turn: a report of the national transgender discrimination survey. National Center for Transgender Equality and National Gay and Lesbian Task Force: Washington; 2011.
12. Edens C. Early sexual health and reproductive implications in pediatric rheumatic diseases. Rheum Dis Clin N Am. 2022;48(1):91–112.
13. Balmuri N, Spitznagle J, Onel K. Patient sexual orientation & gender identity: do you need to know? Ethics forum. Rheumatologist. 2020;
14. Mathias K, Mathias L, Amarnani A, Samko T, Lahita RG, Panush RS. Challenges of caring for transgender and gender diverse patients with rheumatic disease: presentation of seven patients and review of the literature. Curr Opin Rheumatol. 2023;35(2):117–27.
15. LGBTQIA+ Glossary of Terms for Health Care Teams: National LGBTQIA + Health Education Center. 2020. https://www.lgbtqiahealtheducation.org/wp-content/uploads/2020/02/Glossary-2022.02.22-1.pdf. Accessed 26 Apr 2023.
16. Levenson JS, Craig SL, Austin A. Trauma-informed and affirmative mental health practices with LGBTQ+ clients. Psychol Serv. 2023;20:134–44.
17. Invitation to self-identify enhances care of LGBTQ+ patients US: American College of Rheumatology. 2020. https://www.acrconvergencetoday.org/invitation-to-self-identify-enhances-care-of-lgbtq-patients/. Accessed 26 Apr 2023.
18. Healthcare Equality Index 2022 US: The Human Rights Campaign. 2022. https://www.hrc.org/resources/healthcare-equality-index. Accessed 26 Apr 2023.

19. 2015 Edition Health Information Technology (Health IT) Certification Criteria, 2015 Edition Base Electronic Health Record (EHR) Definition, and ONC Health IT Certification Program Modifications. Final rule. Office of the National Coordinator for Health Information Technology (ONC), Department of Health and Human Services (HHS). 2015; 80(200):62601–759.
20. Learning Resources – Publications in Collecting Sexual Orientation and Gender Identity Data US: National LGBTQIA+Health Education Center. 2022. https://www.lgbtqiahealtheducation.org/resources/in/collecting-sexual-orientation-and-gender-identity-data/type/publication/. Accessed 26 Apr 2023.

7 Navigating the Path to Adherence: Fostering Collaborative Patient-Centered Care

Nonadherence in healthcare has emerged as a global problem that spans patient, provider, and healthcare system domains. The issue is further confounded for patients living with chronic illnesses where long-term treatment is often needed for illness management and optimal therapeutic benefit. Adherence and compliance have often been used interchangeably to describe medication-taking behavior among patients. According to the World Health Organization, adherence is "the extent to which a person's behavior – taking medication, following a diet, and/or executing lifestyle changes, corresponds with agreed recommendations from a healthcare provider" [1]. Compliance is defined as "the extent to which the patient's behavior matches the prescriber's recommendations" [2]. There is overwhelming evidence related to the value of patient input and partnership in creating appropriate treatment plans to achieve the best care outcomes. Over the years, adherence has been recognized as the most appropriate term, acknowledging how critical the patient-provider partnership is in making and following through with healthcare decisions. Taking into consideration the patient's beliefs, personal circumstances, experiences, support systems, and available resources is key to optimizing the care plan. This perspective puts the patient at the center of care, where providers and patients intentionally discuss care plans and come to a conclusion that is respected even if it's not in line with the provider's recommendations [2].

J. Rose-Smith et al., *The Psychosocial Impact of Rheumatic Conditions*, https://doi.org/10.1007/978-3-031-95338-5_7

The World Health Organization (WHO) reported that adherence to long-term therapy was poor across various chronic illnesses and severely negatively impacted the quality of life, safety, and healthcare costs [1].

Research shows that poor adherence increases the cost of already high medical interventions, hospitalizations, and physician visits [3]. Research indicates that rheumatoid arthritis affects approximately 1% of the population, a number that continues to rise, making it one of the most prevalent musculoskeletal disorders. Although studies show that RA can be successfully treated, when insufficiently treated, it can result in detrimental joint damage and reduction in function and quality of life. Poor adherence to RA medication is a big barrier to effective illness management. Studies show that adherence to RA medications is low, often resulting in worsening illness and unnecessarily high levels of disease activity, and compromised function in the joints affected [4]. An overview of the current literature on adherence in rheumatic illnesses found that it varied significantly, between 9.3% and 94%, depending on the rheumatic disease [3].

Research describes two kinds of adherence behavior: intentional nonadherence and unintentional nonadherence. Intentional nonadherence is based on a patient's own decision to discontinue medical intervention. This can be influenced by several factors, including adverse side effects, little improvement in condition, and the patient's own belief in poor patient-provider interpersonal factors [4, 5]. Unintentional nonadherence is based on circumstances outside of the patient's control or influence, including costs, health literacy, patient forgetfulness, and complex regiments [4]. The WHO identified five factors that influence nonadherence: socioeconomic factors, healthcare system factors, condition-related factors, therapy-related factors, and patient-related factors [1, 6].

Socioeconomic Factors

Research shows that 43% of working-age adults were inadequately insured in 2022. These individuals were uninsured (9%), had a gap in coverage over the past year (11%), or were insured all year but were underinsured, meaning that their coverage didn't provide them with affordable access to healthcare (23%). Minority Americans were disproportionality represented in this group [7]. In 2021 the official poverty rate in the USA was 11.6%, with 37.9 million people in poverty [8]. The financial burden of managing a chronic illness is a barrier to adherence to medical regimens. One study showed that patients with RA having out-of-pocket costs above $50 per week dropped follow-up visits by 25% compared to patients with out-of-pocket costs below $50/week [9]. Another study found that nearly 70% of patients cannot comply with prescribed medication due to limited financial resources [4]. Older adults are especially impacted by the out-of-pocket cost of medications and often forgo basic needs in order to pay for medications because the condition is expensive to treat and may also result in underemployment or work disability [10].

Communication about the cost of RA drugs was found to be lacking in one study, where rheumatologists were found to discuss medication costs in only one-third of visits where drug therapy was being changed; also, the study found that communication about medication costs was less frequent in non-White and low-income patients [11].

Healthcare System Factors

Appropriate access to care is one of the primary issues contributing to nonadherence. This issue disproportionately impacts minority patients and those impacted by low socioeconomic status. These populations often experience issues with navigating the health system, financial challenges in paying for medication co-pays and expensive therapies not covered by insurance, and timely appointments and communication with their physicians [6]. Transportation and challenges in scheduling follow-up appointments were found to be factors impacting patient's adherence to healthcare recommendations in a study of RA and lupus patients with low socioeconomic status [6]. Other factors related to the healthcare system were agreed upon by experts: short duration of care time per patient and infrequent and low-intensity patient follow-up were also well documented in the literature [12].

Physician Factors

The patient-provider relationship is key to optimizing care, especially for patients with rheumatic illnesses. Research shows that a poor patient-provider relationship is a key factor in predicting nonadherence. This includes several factors, such as low confidence in the healthcare professional, a lack of patient participation in the decision-making process, poor satisfaction with the consultation, and a lack of communication between the patient and provider [12]. Other studies also found that medical and social support was significantly correlated with adherence, which suggests that a supportive environment may improve adherence [13]. Another study with lupus patients showed that patients were least adherent when physicians did not include what they valued as a part of the treatment plan; physicians were perceived to be focused on preventing organ damage and death, and less than 10% of respondents cited these long-term impacts as reasons for adherence [14].

Significant racial disparities have also been found in nonadherence literature; one study with SLE patients shows that African Americans had lower adherence rates. This was associated with perceiving fewer "compassionate, respectful" interactions with providers and worse anxiety and negative affect demonstrated by providers. However, in that study, among White patients, lower adherence was only associated with a higher SLE medication regimen burden and fibromyalgia pain score [15].

Patient-Related Factors

The psychosocial impact of having a chronic illness is well documented in the literature. The onset of symptoms, the unpredictability of the prognosis, the complexity of illness management, often delayed diagnosis, and loss of control often cause emotional distress [16]. Depression is one of the most common mental illnesses reported by patients with rheumatic conditions; major depression and anxiety were prominently associated with medical nonadherence in RA patients in several studies [12, 17–19]. A study examining the impact of depression on medication nonadherence uncovered that patients suffering from depression reported a 2.3-fold increased rate of medication nonadherence than nondepressed patients [20].

Patient understanding of illness and treatment is also critical to adherence. Patients who had a greater understanding of their illness pathology and were educated about the impact of treatment were more likely to be adherent; this issue can impact self-efficacy and patient confidence in managing their illness [12].

Research also found that poor lifestyle behaviors, such as smoking, were associated with poor adherence [12]. Another key reason for nonadherence is higher patient-physician discordance leading to decreased patient satisfaction. Studies report that 40–60% of patients could not correctly report what their physicians expected of them 10–80 min after they were provided with the information. Yet another study reported that over 60% of patients interviewed immediately after visiting their doctors misunderstood the directions regarding prescribed medications [21]. Health literacy refers to the ability to acquire, comprehend, and pursue health information to guide health-related decisions. One major factor that influences adherence is the patient's ability to read and understand medication instructions. Patients with low literacy may have difficulty understanding instructions; this ultimately results in decreased adherence and poor medication management [21].

Condition-Related Factors and Therapy-Related Factors

Complex medication regimens are often a reality for many chronically ill patients. Poor adherence is linked to the complexity of medication regimens, which could include improper timing of drug administration or administration of numerous medications at frequent or unusual times during the day [21]. Studies have shown that less frequent drug dosing resulted in high adherence, while frequent dosing throughout the day was associated with poorer adherence [22]. A cross-sectional study assessing the common reasons for methotrexate adherence in RA found that a lack of understanding of how the medication works leads to nonadherence. The slow-acting potential of the drug was not thoroughly explained, and the patients lost confidence in the drug's ability to be affected. This experience was being compared with other drugs such as corticosteroids, which are more fast-acting; this caused nonadherence [23]. Adverse side effects are another therapy-related factor in nonadherence across rheumatic illnesses [24].

In one study with RA patients, common reasons for nonadherence were related to unintentional adherence factors such as forgetting to take medications; hectic work schedules; household responsibilities, such as errands; and reports about complicated treatment regimens and running out of medications. These issues were further deepened by comorbidities and the management of other illnesses [21].

Strategies to Address Adherence

A team approach is needed for addressing and mitigating factors driving nonadherence and its impacts on patient care and health outcomes. Patients, health systems, providers, and government systems related to insurance access all have a part to play in coming up with viable frameworks, policies, and interventions to improve adherence and, ultimately, the overall health of the patient. Below are some strategies to consider [21]:

- **Partner with Patients**
  - Engage patients in partnership early in the patient-provider relationship by involving them in small and large decisions related to their overall healthcare.
  - Take the time to get to know the patient, do not make assumptions, and treat each patient as an individual; and avoid lumping patients into categories which can put you at risk for stereotyping and bias.
  - Ask about what's valuable to them to learn about who they are and what motivates them in pursuing care and treatment.

- Specify a role for patients when creating the treatment plan, asking them to provide goals and walk you through how they plan to achieve those goals.
- Ask about what you can do to help them achieve their healthcare goals.
- Create a plan to check in, especially if there are long gaps between appointments, to ensure you are communicating about changes, adverse side effects, medication effectiveness, or other changing circumstances in the patient's life.
- Ask about who supports them and if they would like a caregiver or loved one involved in their care.
- Consider using shared decision-making techniques (see Chap. 4).

• **Provide Patient Education**
  - Assess the way that your patients best learn and communicate with them in that way to enhance understanding of treatment and the overall care plan.
  - Explain the *what*, *why*, *when*, *how*, and *duration* of the medications or interventions being prescribed.
  - Spend time discussing side effects or possible adverse reactions, and explain thoroughly the difference between a common side effect that doesn't need medical attention and one that they should consider an emergency. Create a plan for how to handle emergency situations related to treatment.
  - Use the teach-back method to assess understanding of information (see Chap. 4).
  - Use visual decision aids; this can help with patients who have low literacy, including low health literacy, as well as help those with low language proficiency.
  - Educate patients about treatment and care interventions in their own language.
  - Send patients home with written or verbal instructions, including visuals that allow them to clearly remember the regimen.
  - Use tools such as pill boxes, treatment management digital apps with reminders for dosage, and time for taking medications, as well as pill count features.

- **Simplify Treatment Plan/Regimen**
  - Seek to understand the patient's medical care picture and the various treatment and care interventions the patient is following.
  - Consider the easiest treatment uptake for the patient as appropriate.
  - Simplify dosage and frequency of medication.
  - Discuss medication interactions.
  - Encourage the patient to connect with the pharmacist to create another level of support for addressing questions and concerns about the treatment.
- **Consider Social Determinants of Health**
  - Initiate a discussion about the patient's ability to afford treatment.
  - Assess insurance access and financial resources available for copays or other out-of-pocket costs.
  - Ask patients if they have any barriers to transportation, childcare, food, and housing insecurity.
  - Assess for abuse and safety concerns in the home.
  - Consider neighborhood safety and other resources available to the patient before recommending lifestyle/behavior changes around diet, exercises, etc.
- **Discuss Mental Health**
  - Normalize discussions around feelings of distress, depression, anxiety, or other mental health concerns throughout the care relationship.
  - Work with other team members such as social workers, nurses, and other community agencies to provide ongoing support and referrals for patients dealing with these challenges.
- **Other Considerations**
  - Encourage patients when they are doing well, call out positive behaviors, and reinforce creative solutions that yield success.
  - Use empathy with patients; avoid blaming and condemning.

- Assess for adherence during follow-up appointments, check with their pharmacy for treatment pickup, and ask the patient to share their routine with you.
- Review the patient's understanding of the care plan and treatment recommendations.
- Check-in to see if patients had any adverse side effects.
- Encourage patients to bring a family member or loved one to the appointment and engage that support person.
- Use your power and influence to write letters to insurance companies and local and national government bodies to support improved access to care (e.g., insurance access).

References

1. Sabaté E. Adherence to long-term therapies: evidence for action. World Health Organization; 2003.
2. Chakrabarti S. What's in a name? Compliance, adherence, and concordance in chronic psychiatric disorders. World J Psychiatry. 2014;4(2):30–6.
3. Anghel LA, Farcaş AM, Oprean RN. Medication adherence and persistence in patients with autoimmune rheumatic diseases: a narrative review. Patient Prefer Adherence. 2018;12:1151–66.
4. Chowdhury T, Dutta J, Noel P, Islam R, Gonzalez-Peltier G, Azad S, et al. An overview on causes of nonadherence in the treatment of rheumatoid arthritis: its effect on mortality and ways to improve adherence. Cureus. 2022;14(4)
5. Balsa A, de Yébenes MJG, Carmona L. Multilevel factors predict medication adherence in rheumatoid arthritis: a 6-month cohort study. Ann Rheum Dis. 2022;81(3):327–34.
6. Marengo MF, Suarez-Almazor ME. Improving treatment adherence in patients with rheumatoid arthritis: what are the options? Int J Clin Rheumtol. 2015;10(5):345–56.
7. Collins SR, Haynes LA, Masitha R. The state of US health insurance in 2022: findings from the Commonwealth Fund biennial health insurance survey. The Commonwealth Fund. 2022;29.
8. National Poverty in America Awareness Month: 2022. Report No.: P60–277.
9. Curkendall S, Patel V, Gleeson M, Campbell RS, Zagari M, Dubois R. Compliance with biologic therapies for rheumatoid arthritis: do patient out-of-pocket payments matter? Arthritis Rheum. 2008;59(10):1519–26.

10. Harrold LR, Briesacher BA, Peterson D, Beard A, Madden J, Zhang F, et al. Cost-related medication nonadherence in older patients with rheumatoid arthritis. J Rheumatol. 2013;40(2):137–43.
11. Beard AJ, Sleath B, Blalock SJ, Roth M, Weinberger M, Tudor G, et al. Predictors of rheumatoid arthritis patient-physician communication about medication costs during visits to rheumatologists. Arthritis Care Res (Hoboken). 2010;62(5):632–9.
12. Gil-Guillen VF, Balsa A, Bernárdez B, Valdés YLC, Márquez-Contreras E, de la Haba-Rodríguez J, et al. Medication non-adherence in rheumatology, oncology and cardiology: a review of the literature of risk factors and potential interventions. Int J Environ Res Public Health. 2022;19(19)
13. Betegnie AL, Gauchet A, Lehmann A, Grange L, Roustit M, Baudrant M, et al. Why do patients with chronic inflammatory rheumatic diseases discontinue their biologics? An assessment of patients' adherence using a self-report questionnaire. J Rheumatol. 2016;43(4):724–30.
14. Sloan M, Lever E, Gordon C, Harwood R, Georgopoulou S, Naughton F, et al. Medication decision-making and adherence in lupus: patient-physician discordance and the impact of previous 'adverse medical experiences'. Rheumatology (Oxford). 2022;61(4):1417–29.
15. Sun K, Eudy AM, Criscione-Schreiber LG, Sadun RE, Rogers JL, Doss J, et al. Racial disparities in medication adherence between African American and Caucasian patients with systemic lupus erythematosus and their associated factors. ACR Open Rheumatol. 2020;2(7):430–7.
16. Geenen R, Newman S, Bossema ER, Vriezekolk JE, Boelen PA. Psychological interventions for patients with rheumatic diseases and anxiety or depression. Best Pract Res Clin Rheumatol. 2012;26(3):305–19.
17. Santiago T, Geenen R, Jacobs JW, Da Silva JA. Psychological factors associated with response to treatment in rheumatoid arthritis. Curr Pharm Des. 2015;21(2):257–69.
18. Matcham F, Rayner L, Steer S, Hotopf M. The prevalence of depression in rheumatoid arthritis: a systematic review and meta-analysis. Rheumatology (Oxford). 2013;52(12):2136–48.
19. Arturi P, Schneeberger EE, Sommerfleck F, Buschiazzo E, Ledesma C, Maldonado Cocco JA, et al. Adherence to treatment in patients with ankylosing spondylitis. Clin Rheumatol. 2013;32(7):1007–15.
20. Goh H, Kwan YH, Seah Y, Low LL, Fong W, Thumboo J. A systematic review of the barriers affecting medication adherence in patients with rheumatic diseases. Rheumatol Int. 2017;37(10):1619–28.
21. Jimmy B, Jose J. Patient medication adherence: measures in daily practice. Oman Med J. 2011;26(3):155–9.
22. van den Bemt BJ, Zwikker HE, van den Ende CH. Medication adherence in patients with rheumatoid arthritis: a critical appraisal of the existing literature. Expert Rev Clin Immunol. 2012;8(4):337–51.

23. Alrubaye YS, Al-Juboori B, Al-Humairi AK. The causes of non-adherence to methotrexate in patients with rheumatoid arthritis. Res J Pharm Technol. 2021;14(2):769–74.
24. Hope HF, Hyrich KL, Anderson J, Bluett J, Sergeant JC, Barton A, et al. The predictors of and reasons for non-adherence in an observational cohort of patients with rheumatoid arthritis commencing methotrexate. Rheumatology (Oxford). 2020;59(1):213–23.

Using a Team Approach to Achieve Optimal Outcomes

8

Managing rheumatic illnesses in patients requires a team effort. The American College of Rheumatology (ACR) and the European League Against Rheumatism (EULAR) both recognize the importance of team-based care in managing patients with rheumatic diseases. While they may not have a single, unified set of guidelines specifically focused explicitly on team-based care, both organizations emphasize the interprofessional approach as a core component of effective rheumatologic care. The ACR guidelines emphasize that multidisciplinary care is a critical component in the management of patients with rheumatic diseases, particularly those with complex or multisystem involvement. The EULAR also places significant emphasis on a holistic, interdisciplinary approach to managing rheumatic diseases, especially in conditions such as rheumatoid arthritis, psoriatic arthritis, lupus, and other inflammatory arthritis and autoimmune diseases [1, 2]. (American College of Rheumatology. [2019]. *Position Statement on Interdisciplinary Teams in Rheumatology).*

The literature underscores that team-based care is critical to ensuring that all members of the healthcare team are aligned with the patient's goals, the treatment objectives, and the specific roles each provider plays in achieving these outcomes. Effective communication and coordination among team members—whether they are physicians, nurses, social workers, physical therapists, specialists, or nonclinical professionals—are essential for

J. Rose-Smith et al., *The Psychosocial Impact of Rheumatic Conditions*, https://doi.org/10.1007/978-3-031-95338-5_8

delivering safe, high-quality care. By working collaboratively and in concert, these professionals are able to provide comprehensive, patient-centered care that meets the complex needs of the individual [3–5].

> I saw six providers in the past two weeks and came away with nineteen different medicines, did the same test three times and I am still confused about the plan. –Lupus Patient

Through effective communication and a well-defined collaborative framework, healthcare providers can reduce duplication of treatment interventions and diagnostic tests, enhance clarity in treatment pathways, minimize errors, and mitigate other forms of medical waste within the system. This collaborative approach not only improves the efficiency of care but also contributes to better patient outcomes and higher levels of patient satisfaction [6, 7].

It is not sufficient to simply refer to a group of healthcare providers as a "team." For effective interprofessional collaboration, the team must formally recognize themselves as a cohesive unit. This involves identifying shared goals, establishing clear communication pathways, and making treatment decisions tailored to the individual patient. The team must also implement a unified method for exchanging information across healthcare settings and ensure that the patient's and their caregivers' voices are integral to the care process. Regular team meetings are essential for reviewing and adjusting care plans in alignment with the patient's evolving needs and preferences. By grounding care in the patient's values and continuously aligning treatment strategies with their goals, the team ensures that the care provided is both comprehensive and patient-centered [6].

Today, tools such as electronic medical records (EMRs) and systems like Care Everywhere, which facilitate the seamless sharing of patient information, enable healthcare providers to more easily view and collaborate on the care plans established by other team members. In addition, virtual meetings and other digital technologies enable teams to engage with both patients and each other in real time, enhancing communication and coordination [8]. These platforms foster meaningful interactions, clarify roles within the team, and ensure that patient preferences are incorporated into the care plan, ultimately improving collaboration. Team-based care also offers opportunities to optimize patient engagement through strategies like shared decision-making, which strengthens the patient-provider partnership, builds trust, and leads to increased patient satisfaction [9, 10].

Barriers to Team-Based Care

Implementing team-based care can be challenging. Like other healthcare providers, rheumatology providers can face significant barriers when trying to implement team-based care for patients with chronic conditions. Taking steps at both the individual and system levels to overcome these barriers proactively is important in overcoming some of the challenges of team-based care.

- **Fragmented and siloed healthcare delivery system:** In many healthcare systems, professionals such as physicians, nurses, physical therapists, specialists, social workers, and researchers often work in silos, which can create significant barriers to effective collaboration. Physicians and healthcare organizations frequently face challenges related to limited access to key healthcare professionals, including primary care providers, nurses, and social workers. These workforce shortages complicate the development of comprehensive, fully functional multidisciplinary teams. As a result, the responsibility of care coordination often falls disproportionately on the rheumatologist or a small number of team members, leading to frustration, burnout, and an imbalance in workload distribution and compensation [11–15].
- **Lack of shared electronic health records (EHRs) and digital tools:** Electronic health records have revolutionized communicating across teams and care systems for many in healthcare. However, we continue to be challenged by poor integration of EHRs across systems and individual providers, which can lead to gaps in communication, duplication, and inefficiencies due to lack of access to test results, diagnosis,

treatment plan, psychosocial concerns, and overall care team notes [16, 17].

- **Lack of resources to assist in coordinating care:** The role of care coordinators or a clearly defined care coordination function is often not formally established within healthcare teams. When care coordination is necessary, it is frequently assumed by individual providers or a small group of professionals, driven by their personal interest in ensuring comprehensive care. This often leads to ambiguity in roles and responsibilities, resulting in confusion, duplication of efforts, or gaps in care. In multidisciplinary teams, professionals from different healthcare systems or disciplines may take on overlapping responsibilities and adopt divergent approaches to care or collaboration, which can create more challenges than solutions. Additionally, many healthcare providers are not adequately trained in collaborative care or team-based approaches, limiting the effectiveness of interprofessional teams due to insufficient communication and coordination and hindering overall team performance [18, 19].
- **Limited time:** Time is a limited resource in healthcare, and team-based care requires providers to dedicate time for case discussions, treatment plan coordination, and follow-up, which can be perceived as impractical. With increasing patient volumes and reimbursement constraints, the demands of individual care often take precedence, making it challenging to prioritize collaborative care efforts [6].
- **Reimbursement models:** Although some payment models incentivize team-based care, the majority of reimbursement structures in healthcare continue to prioritize individual care and consultations. Additionally, policies and regulations governing scope of practice, licensure, and reimbursement can limit the roles and contributions of providers across the interprofessional team. These constraints may create disincentives or hinder the full potential of interdisciplinary teams, ultimately restricting their effectiveness in delivering coordinated, comprehensive care [20, 21].

- **Communication:** Effective communication is the cornerstone of team-based care. When team members do not communicate effectively or fail to share critical information, it can lead to errors, delays in care, and poor patient outcomes. Barriers to communication can include physical distance between team members, lack of technology to facilitate effective communication, lack of standardized communication protocols, or differences in professional language, terminology, and care philosophy. Additionally, differences in professional culture and power dynamics can cause misunderstanding between team members and impede collaboration and care [22, 23].
- **Patient preferences and engagement:** Some patients may prefer a single provider or find it difficult to navigate the complexity of a team-based approach. This can be particularly true for patients with chronic conditions who are accustomed to seeing the same provider for all their needs. Engaging patients in a team-based care model requires educating them about the benefits of this approach and overcoming any hesitation they may have [24].
- **Complexity of chronic illness:** Rheumatic illnesses can be very complex, requiring extensive care coordination across teams and health systems. This can be daunting for providers and patients, causing disengagement for patients and providers. For team-based care to be effective, it is essential that both patients and providers understand its benefits and are fully committed to the collaborative approach [11].

How to Optimize Team-Based Care

- **Support infrastructure and structural system changes:** Rheumatology providers can work with healthcare organizations to demonstrate the value of team-based care by establishing or enhancing care coordination roles within the team. For example, a nurse care coordinator or social worker who specializes in rheumatology can help facilitate communication between team members and ensure that patients are receiving coordinated care across disciplines [25].

- **Exploring various value-based payment models:** Although value-based care arrangements are continuing to emerge and become more popular, rheumatology professionals can continue to advocate—through ACR and other bodies—for policy changes that support reimbursement for team-based care. Bundle payments, shared savings programs, and other strategies help to incentivize providers across the care continuum so they engage in collaboration. Providers can lobby for these kinds of payment models. The goal is to improve provider motivation for engagement in this best practice of team-based care. In the current system, rheumatology providers can work within their system to explore and optimize the use of existing models—such as chronic care management codes and other billing codes, and care coordination services—to fund team-based care. Partnering with community organizations or interested donors to provide pilot funding for team-based care is also a good place to start to demonstrate the effectiveness of this approach and its many benefits, especially in enhancing patient care, safety, satisfaction, and outcomes [8].
- **Leverage telehealth and use digital tools:** Rheumatology professionals can advocate for better integration of care across specialties by promoting the use of shared electronic health records (EHRs) and fostering seamless communication between providers. Enhanced data sharing can improve care coordination and help break down silos across teams and healthcare systems. Additionally, telemedicine and other digital tools can be leveraged to facilitate efficient collaboration with providers and key team members both within and outside the healthcare system, supporting the patient's care plan. Telehealth also improves access to the interprofessional team, particularly in rural or underserved areas, where patients may face barriers to in-person consultations [8].
- **Create/identify care coordination roles:** Many providers and healthcare systems are contending with resource constraint and may not be able to invest in dedicated coordinator roles; however, to address this, collaborative care training can be supported by rheumatology providers. These training opportunities can bring together professionals from different disciplines.

Joint seminars, workshops, or simulation-based training focused on teamwork, communication, and the nuances of managing chronic rheumatic diseases can be focus areas from which the interprofessional team can benefit. Additionally, encouraging cross-training for different care team members such as nurses, physical therapists, social workers, and occupational therapists can provide a better understanding of each team member's roles to avoid duplication and build some cross-coverage as appropriate [26].

- **Nurture collaboration as part of the culture:** In many healthcare settings, individual autonomy and a hierarchical culture exist; however, rheumatology providers can actively promote a collaborative mindset within their practices by encouraging open communication, mutual respect, and shared decision-making among all team members. By modeling collaborative behaviors, rheumatology providers can help build trust and break down hierarchical barriers [22].
- **Structure collaborative communication:** Part of successfully establishing team-based care is standardizing communication protocols, such as regular interdisciplinary case conferences or structured handoff procedures. These can ensure that all team members are on the same page. Regular in-person or virtual rounds should be established to ensure everyone is kept updated on the progress of the treatment plan, discuss challenges, and provide opportunities for each team member to contribute ideas and revise the plan as appropriate. Additionally, EHRs should be used to share updated notes, test results, and other critical clinical and psychosocial information. This ensures that all team members have real-time access to all information to better support the patient. The interprofessional team should also ensure they clarify roles and responsibilities to avoid role ambiguity—it's essential to clearly define the scope of practice and responsibilities of each team member [27–29].
- **Creating time:** Time constraints are a common challenge in healthcare, but these can be mitigated by optimizing workflows and processes that allow providers to delegate tasks such as routine follow-ups, patient education, prescription updates, and coordination of team meetings. Nurse practitioners, nurses,

social workers, and physician assistants can take on these responsibilities, thus freeing up time for the rheumatologist to focus on more complex aspects of patient care. Proper delegation not only reduces administrative burdens but also improves scheduling efficiency, allowing for more time dedicated to collaboration with other team members. Additionally, digital health tools, such as telehealth platforms and remote monitoring devices, can assist rheumatologists in managing patient care outside of traditional office visits. These technologies enable ongoing care management, help track disease progression, and facilitate communication with patients, further enhancing the time available for intensive team-based collaboration when needed [6, 30, 31].

- **Fostering mutual respect and a collaborative culture:** Rheumatology providers can foster an environment that values the contributions of all team members, regardless of their professional titles. By encouraging open dialogue, cultivating a nonhierarchical atmosphere, and respecting each professional's expertise, rheumatologists—along with other team members who are perceived to hold more authority—can help reduce barriers created by hierarchical structures. This approach sets the expectation for a culture of collaboration. Additionally, promoting mutual respect among team members is essential for optimizing the team's overall effectiveness. Rheumatologists can demonstrate respect for the expertise of other professionals, such as physical therapists, dietitians, and social workers, thereby promoting a culture where interdisciplinary collaboration is not only valued but recognized as critical to delivering high-quality patient care [32–34].
- **Patient-centered care:** Patient education is essential in helping both patients and their caregivers understand the benefits of team-based care. Rheumatologists and rheumatology professionals play a critical role in educating patients about who is involved in the care team and how the interprofessional team will provide comprehensive care—including mental health support, physical therapy, and connections to community resources as needed. These discussions can also highlight why a collaborative, team-based approach is the most effective way to manage the patient's care, ensuring that the responsibility

for coordinating care does not fall solely on the patient. When creating the treatment plan, a team-based approach enables the incorporation of the patient's goals and preferences, utilizing tools like shared decision-making, the teach-back method, and the Ask Me 3® model to facilitate meaningful patient engagement (See Chap. 10, p. 102 for details) [35]. Furthermore, this approach allows for the optimization of contributions from other team members, such as nutritionists, social workers, and physical therapists, which enhances buy-in from both the care team and the patient. As a result, the emerging care plan is more likely to reflect the patient's goals, values, and social context, ensuring it is both effective and person-centered [36–40].

- **Use community resources:** Individual rheumatology care providers and some healthcare systems have limited resources and often no access to providers such as social workers, care navigators, physical therapists, nutritionists, or mental health providers. Community resources such as support groups, mental health organizations, and social organizations can provide patients with emotional and psychosocial support. These resources can complement a patient's care plan by helping patients manage the emotional impact of chronic illness, build coping skills, optimize self-management, and reduce feelings of isolation and fear. Rheumatology teams can work with social workers, care coordinators, or patient navigators outside of their practices or healthcare systems to connect patients to these resources. Patients can face huge financial challenges when managing a chronic rheumatic illness, which often requires ongoing treatment that can be financially burdensome even with insurance. Community organizations often have financial assistance programs that can help supplement the cost of care and medical equipment or pharmacy discount programs. Illness-specific or charitable organizations can help reduce the financial strain on patients. Transportation can be a significant barrier to accessing care as well as other social determinants of health challenges. The rheumatologist, social workers, nurses, and care coordinators can assist in navigating key community resources that can help support patients in addressing these important needs.

Psychological Safety: Speak Up!

According to the Harvard Business review, psychological safety "is a shared belief held by members of a team that it's OK to take risks, to express their ideas and concerns, to speak up with questions, and to admit mistakes—all without fear of negative consequences" [41]. Psychological safety has emerged as an important catalyst for high-level team performance [42]. However, in some healthcare settings, a traditional hierarchy exists where physicians are viewed as the primary decision-makers. This hierarchy can hinder collaborative decision-making, discourage input from other team members, and create power imbalances that undermine the effectiveness of team-based care. Rheumatologists and other care providers can help create an environment that values input from all team members, regardless of their professional title, by encouraging open dialogue, creating a nonhierarchical atmosphere. By valuing each professional's expertise, rheumatologists can reduce barriers created by hierarchical structures.

Encouraging mutual respect between team members is essential to fostering psychological safety in a team-based care model. This can "lead to better decision-making, as people feel more comfortable voicing their opinions and concerns, which often leads to a more diverse range of perspectives being heard and considered" [41]. Rheumatologists can demonstrate respect for the expertise of other team members, such as physical therapists, dietitians, or social workers, promoting a culture where interdisciplinary collaboration is valued and essential to patient care.

Conclusion

As healthcare systems evolve, it will be essential to create environments that facilitate and incentivize team-based care to optimize the management of patients with chronic complex rheumatic illness. Rheumatology professionals need to work to address barriers to team-based care through proactive leadership, advocacy for structural and systems change, improved communication, optimizing technology, and fostering a culture of collaboration. By doing so rheumatologists and rheumatology professionals can overcome many of the challenges associated with team-based care. The evidence shows that team-based care can optimize patient outcomes, satisfaction, quality of care, and overall experience, helping healthcare systems and individuals to avoid medical errors and reduce waste. Rheumatologists play a pivotal role in leading and coordinating these teams, ensuring that patients with chronic conditions receive comprehensive, coordinated care. With thoughtful planning, advocacy, and interprofessional collaboration, rheumatologists can enhance the effectiveness of team-based care and significantly improve outcomes for patients with chronic rheumatic conditions.

References

1. American College of Rheumatology. Interdisciplinary care team. 2023. Available from: https://rheumatology.org/interdisciplinary-care-team
2. Smolen JS, Landewé RBM, Bijlsma JWJ, Burmester GR, Dougados M, Kerschbaumer A, et al. EULAR recommendations for the management of rheumatoid arthritis with synthetic and biological disease-modifying antirheumatic drugs: 2019 update. Ann Rheum Dis. 2020;79(6):685–99.
3. Wagner EH. The role of patient care teams in chronic disease management. BMJ. 2000;320(7234):569–72.
4. Cadet T, Cusimano J, McKearney S, Honaker J, O'Neal C, Taheri R, et al. Describing the evidence linking interprofessional education interventions to improving the delivery of safe and effective patient care: a scoping review. J Interprof Care. 2024;38(3):476–85.
5. Steinbarger K. The Rheumatologist®. 2024. Make Way for the Interprofessional Rheumatology Team! Available from: https://www.the-rheumatologist.org/article/make-way-for-the-interprofessional-rheumatology-team/
6. Smith CD, Balatbat C, Corbridge S, Dopp AL, Fried J, Harter R, et al. Implementing optimal team-based care to reduce clinician burnout. Nam Perspect. 2018;8(9):1–13.
7. Zajac S, Woods A, Tannenbaum S, Salas E, Holladay CL. Overcoming challenges to teamwork in healthcare: a team effectiveness framework and evidence-based guidance. Front Commun. 2021;6:606445.
8. O'Malley AS, Draper K, Gourevitch R, Cross DA, Scholle SH. Electronic health records and support for primary care teamwork. J Am Med Inform Assoc. 2015;22(2):426–34.

9. Elwyn G, Frosch DL, Kobrin S. Implementing shared decision-making: consider all the consequences. Implement Sci. 2016;11:114.
10. Street RLJ, Makoul G, Arora NK, Epstein RM. How does communication heal? Pathways linking clinician-patient communication to health outcomes. Patient Educ Couns. 2009;74(3):295–301.
11. Montano AR, Cornell PY, Gravenstein S. Barriers and facilitators to interprofessional collaborative practice for community-dwelling older adults: an integrative review. J Clin Nurs. 2023;32(9–10):1534–48.
12. Brooks L, Elliott J, Stolee P, Boscart VM, Gimbel S, Holisek B, et al. Development, successes, and potential pitfalls of multidisciplinary chronic disease management clinics in a family health team: a qualitative study. BMC Prim Care. 2023;24(1):126. https://doi.org/10.1186/s12875-023-02073-x.
13. Duda-Sikuła M, Kurpas D. Barriers and facilitators in the implementation of prevention strategies for chronic disease patients-best practice guidelines and policies' systematic review. J Pers Med. 2023;13(2):288.
14. American Hospital Association. Legal (Fraud and Abuse) Barriers To Care Transformation and How to Address Them [Internet]. American Hospital Association. 2017. Available from: https://www.aha.org/system/files/content/16/barrierstocare-full.pdf
15. Martin P, Pighills A, Burge V, Argus G, Sinclair L. Promoting Interprofessional education and collaborative practice in rural health settings: learnings from a state-wide multi-methods study. Int J Environ Res Public Health. 2021;18(10)
16. Vos JFJ, Boonstra A, Kooistra A, Seelen M, van Offenbeek M. The influence of electronic health record use on collaboration among medical specialties. BMC Health Serv Res. 2020;20(1):676.
17. Robertson ST, Rosbergen ICM, Burton-Jones A, Grimley RS, Brauer SG. The effect of the electronic health record on interprofessional practice: a systematic review. Appl Clin Inform. 2022;13(3):541–59.
18. Zwarenstein M, Goldman J, Reeves S. Interprofessional collaboration: effects of practice-based interventions on professional practice and healthcare outcomes. Cochrane Database Syst Rev. 2009;6(3):CD000072.
19. Reeves S, Pelone F, Harrison R, Goldman J, Zwarenstein M. Interprofessional collaboration to improve professional practice and healthcare outcomes. Cochrane Database Syst Rev. 2017;6(6):CD000072.
20. Khalili H. Transforming health care delivery: innovations in payment models for interprofessional team-based care. N C Med J. 2024;85(3):173–7.
21. Mose JN, Jones CB. Alternative payment models and team-based care. N C Med J. 2018;79(4):231–4.
22. Zajac S, Woods A, Tannenbaum S, Salas E, Holladay CL. Overcoming challenges to teamwork in healthcare: a team effectiveness framework and evidence-based guidance. Front Commun. 2021;6:6.

23. Erjavec K, Knavs N, Bedenčič K. Communication in interprofessional health care teams from the perspective of patients and staff. J Health Sci. 2022;12(1):29–37.
24. Gilchrist Miss R, Kholvadia DA. Patients' perceptions of Interprofessional collaboration: a scoping review. Patient Exp J. 2024;11(1):154–72.
25. Pathak N, Tomolo A, Escoffery C. Improving team-based care coordination delivery and documentation in the health record. Fed Pract. 2018;35(10):32–9.
26. Hempel S, Ganz D, Saluja S, Bolshakova M, Kim T, Turvey C, et al. Care coordination across healthcare systems: development of a research agenda, implications for practice, and recommendations for policy based on a modified Delphi panel. BMJ Open. 2023;13(5):e060232.
27. Apantaku G, Aguiar M, Kaal KJ, Munro S, Teo M, Harrison M. Understanding multidisciplinary care for people with rheumatic disease in British Columbia, Canada, through patients, nurses and physicians voices: a qualitative policy evaluation. BMC Health Serv Res. 2021;21(1):1148.
28. Din BRU, Anjum F, Malik A. Cross-disciplinary collaboration in healthcare: enhancing outcomes through team-based care. Multidiscip J Healthc. 2024;1(1):11–9.
29. Kreps G. Communication and effective interprofessional health care teams. Int Arch Nurs Health Care. 2016;2(3):51.
30. Hopkins K, Sinsky CA. Team-based care: saving time and improving efficiency. Fam Pract Manag. 2014;21(6):23–9.
31. Bers S. How the Cleveland Clinic overcame barriers to team-based care. 2018.
32. Salas E, Zajac S, Marlow SL. Transforming health care one team at a time: ten observations and the trail ahead. Group Organ Manag. 2018;43(3):357–81. https://doi.org/10.1177/1059601118756554.
33. Mitchell P. Core principles and values of effective team-based health care. 2012.
34. Cullati S, Bochatay N, Maître F, Laroche T, Muller-Juge V, Blondon KS, et al. When team conflicts threaten quality of care: a study of health care professionals' experiences and perceptions. Mayo Clin Proc Innov Qual Outcomes. 2019;3(1):43–51.
35. Parcher, J. Supporting Patient-Provider Communication at a Community Mobile Clinic Using the Ask Me Three© Brochure. University of Delaware. 2024.
36. Lorig KR, Mazonson PD, Holman HR. Evidence suggesting that health education for self-management in patients with chronic arthritis has sustained health benefits while reducing health care costs. Arthritis Rheum. 1993;36(4):439–46.
37. Hall J, Julia Kaal K, Lee J, Duncan R, Tsao N, Harrison M. Patient satisfaction and costs of multidisciplinary models of care in rheumatology: a review of the recent literature. Curr Rheumatol Rep. 2018;20(4):19.

38. Kwame A, Petrucka PM. A literature-based study of patient-centered care and communication in nurse-patient interactions: barriers, facilitators, and the way forward. BMC Nurs. 2021;20(1):158.
39. D'Agostino TA, Atkinson TM, Latella LE, Rogers M, Morrissey D, DeRosa AP, et al. Promoting patient participation in healthcare interactions through communication skills training: a systematic review. Patient Educ Couns. 2017;100(7):1247–57.
40. O'Donovan R, McAuliffe E. Exploring psychological safety in healthcare teams to inform the development of interventions: combining observational, survey and interview data. BMC Health Serv Res. 2020;20(1):810.
41. Gallo A. What is psychological safety? Harv Bus Rev. 2023;
42. Castro S, Englmaier F, Guadalupe M. Fostering psychological safety in teams: evidence from an rct. Available SSRN 4141538. 2022.

Engaging the Family and Support System in Patient Care

9

Being diagnosed with a chronic illness not only impacts the patient, but also the entire family. Research shows that family dynamics and routines can be disrupted when a family member develops a chronic illness. Each member of the family experiences their own unique set of challenges. Additionally, evidence reinforces the important role of family and support systems in the coping of individuals living with rheumatic disease. "Rheumatic disease imposes a substantial emotional burden on individuals, leading to chronic pain, discomfort, anxiety, and depression. Coping with unpredictability and physical limitations can create a detrimental feedback loop, exacerbating mental and physical symptoms" [1]. Support networks can help to reduce isolation and depression and increase emotional support in managing the unpredictability of symptoms and psychosocial stressors.

When possible, providers should work to be in active partnership with patients, their families, and support systems to leverage the benefit of creating connections with their patients' support systems beyond the exam room. This can have more influence on how patients care for themselves, understand their illness, and integrate the treatment plan. Research has demonstrated the many benefits of engaging the family and support system in patient care—including improved health outcomes, enhanced patient

J. Rose-Smith et al., *The Psychosocial Impact of Rheumatic Conditions*, https://doi.org/10.1007/978-3-031-95338-5_9

confidence and satisfaction with their treatment plans. Also, there is the benefit of gaining valuable insight into the patient's needs and psychosocial situation, leading to improvements in quality care, overall.

Some of the ways providers can do this include:

- **Encourage shared decision-making**: Invite identified family members or loved ones to participate in discussions around treatment options and potential risks/benefits. It's important to consider the patient and their families' cultural and religious beliefs when choosing the best course of action. Refer to Chap. 4 for more information on shared decision-making.
- **Connect with interdisciplinary colleagues:** Remain in open communication with all team members involved in your patient's care. Connect with social workers, nurses, physical therapists, or other professionals caring for the patient who may be working with family members to address psychosocial barriers to care and may be able to share collateral information and family relationships and dynamics.
- **Collaborate with psychosocial support groups**: Collaborating with psychosocial support groups as an invited speaker or attendee is an opportunity to educate patients and their loved ones around their condition. It also allows physicians and other healthcare professionals to learn from patients and their families' lived experiences, fostering a sense of trust and engagement beyond the exam room.
- **Create patient and family advisory councils**: These forums allow patients and their families to share openly about how to improve healthcare processes for all patients. They also create consistent opportunities to work side by side with patients and families to learn from their perspectives and values. It also provides insight for patients and families on how they may partner with healthcare providers to optimize care delivery [2, 3].

Chronic Illness and the Family Experience: The Pediatric Lens

Family structures can vary widely across cultures, encompassing diverse dynamics. In some cultures, extended family members or community figures may hold significant influence in decision-making processes. When treating the whole patient, it's crucial to recognize and respect these cultural norms, acknowledging that decisions may involve a broader circle of individuals beyond the immediate family. This understanding helps providers ensure comprehensive and culturally responsive care (Fig. 9.1).

Case of Anna

Anna is an 18-year-old Hispanic female diagnosed with SLE since the age of 15. She recently transitioned from pediatric to adult rheumatology and started attending appointments more

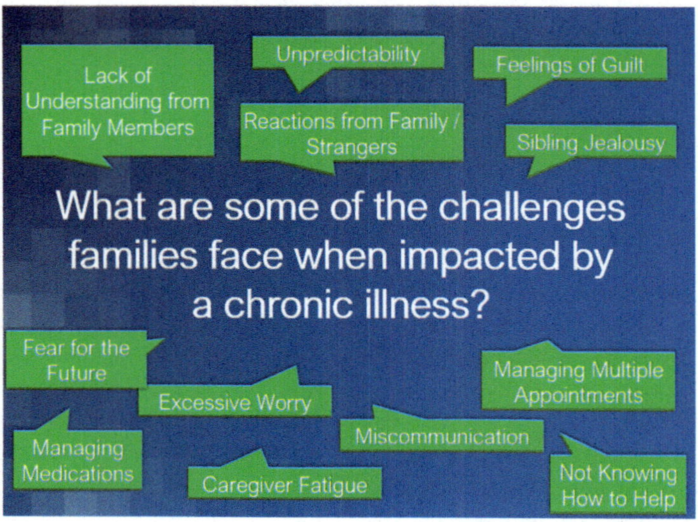

Fig. 9.1 Common challenges experienced by families impacted by chronic illness

independently. Until recently, her mother attended all medical visits and now will often join by phone to listen in. Anna was just discharged from the hospital, following a new diagnosis of lupus nephritis. In a recent follow-up visit, Anna's rheumatologist recommend she begin an IV infusion medication to manage and treat her lupus nephritis. Anna's mother who was listening in on the phone during the visit, immediately states, "No! I don't want her to take any more medications! Why doesn't anyone bother to ask her mother anymore?"

Parents and caregivers, at a different life stage than their child, may cope with the illness differently than their loved ones. Taking care of a child or a loved one comes with a tremendous number of stressors. Some may even be caregivers for a parent, or one may be dealing with a health issue of one's own. When a child receives a diagnosis of a rheumatic disease, it creates new demands on caregivers. Parents or support persons are often the ones who take responsibility for the overall medical management of their child or loved one's healthcare, dealing with their school, multiple absences, and figuring out their work schedule to accommodate appointments. They may also experience different emotions such as fear for the future, anger, and guilt, asking: "Why did this this happen?" These emotions can often manifest themselves in different ways: such as high stress, lack of medical follow-up, anxiety, or depression which is why support is so important. In families where there is more than one child in the home, parents are also balancing the needs of their other children who might behave differently to get more attention.

Thinking back to Anna's case, there were several dynamics at play. Anna is a young adult that is just learning to take ownership of her own healthcare and still relies heavily on her mother to navigate and make important decisions. Despite the patient being of legal age to make medical decisions, Anna's mother feels concerned and protective and remains heavily involved in her child's care. As healthcare providers, how do we intervene to best support our patient in developing self-management skills while also engaging the family in her care?

Providers may consider intervening by fostering open communication with both the young adult and the mother, acknowledging the young adult's growing autonomy while also addressing the mother's concerns. Here are a few communication techniques you may consider to gain an understanding of the patient's and family values around healthcare:

- **Assess family and cultural values around care through open-ended questions:**
  - "Would you like me to include a family member or loved one in this process?"
  - "Please share how medical decisions are made within your family or community."
  - "Are there any specific religious or cultural traditions that influence how you may make decisions around medical treatment or care?"
- **Consider using inviting openers to foster open communication:**
  - "We know that culture and beliefs can often impact how a person thinks, feels, manages and copes with their condition and treatment."
  - "I want to be mindful about how your culture and beliefs may affect your treatment and care."
- **When addressing family members who may be part of a medical visit, it's important to validate family concerns, using statements such as:**
  - "I understand that you are concerned about..."
  - "I can see why that would be a concern" [4].
- **Remember to assess the patient's level of comfort in sharing around sensitive areas of care—even though family members or loved ones may be involved in care, some patients may not want to share all aspects of their medical care—necessitating asking:**
  - "Are you comfortable with me discussing these areas of your care with your loved one?"
  - "What areas of your care that we just discussed would you like me to share with your support system?"

Adolescence is such a vulnerable time to receive a diagnosis of a chronic illness. Tailored interventions are needed to best support patients and families coping with rheumatic conditions.

Adolescence is also a time of many changes—with increased sense of autonomy, among other complex factors, such as negotiating friendship and peer influence. In early adolescence, struggling with one's sense of identity and worrying about being "normal" are common. Looking at our adolescent stages of development, early, middle, and late stages each bring a set of unique challenges. Early on, teens grapple with issues of identity, become less interested in their parents, and are more influenced by their peers. In the middle stage, teens can feel very self-conscious and begin to want more independence. Finally, in late adolescence teens develop a firmer identity, start looking for serious relationships, and become more self-reliant. These are accompanied by several physical changes throughout this time.

When a teen is diagnosed with a chronic illness such as arthritis or lupus, they must cope with many more challenges including the invisible aspects of the disease: "not looking sick," the visible signs such as hair loss, and weight gain/loss from certain medications like steroids or the illness itself. One can experience joint pain which limits one's ability to spend time with friends. Teens also cope with the unpredictability of flares and managing multiple appointments. These factors can disrupt normal adolescent development, which can lead to depression, low self-esteem, and body-image issues. Coping with a chronic illness is in direct conflict with several of the stages of adolescent development [5–7] (Fig. 9.2).

Providers can best support their adolescent patients and families by creating opportunities to engage in peer support. Discuss their interest in speaking individually with another young patient or family coping through a similar experience. Explore their interest in connecting with other community resources, such as a teen-specific support groups, which create safe spaces to share about developmental concerns specific to living with a chronic illness such as body image, dating, or communicating with friends or loved ones about lupus. These opportunities to connect will also allow parents to learn new skills to support their children.

One example of tailored support for adolescents and their families living with lupus is the Charla de Lupus (Lupus Chat)® Program which offers bicultural support to patients with lupus and their families.

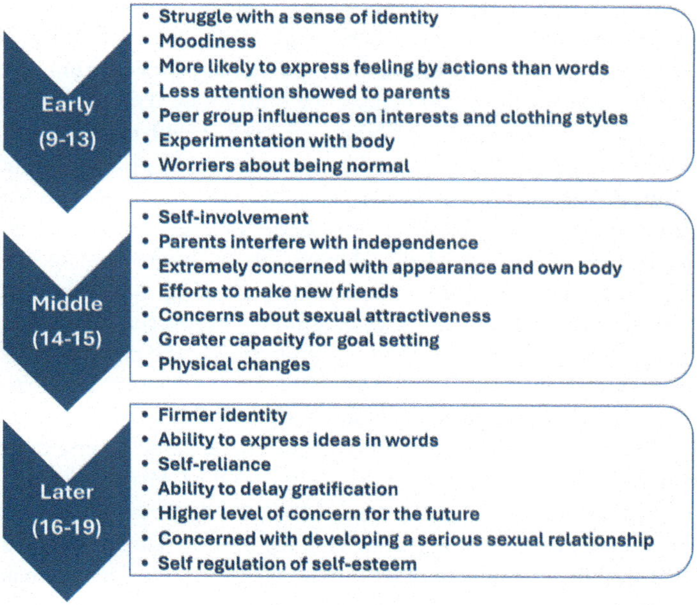

Fig. 9.2 Stages of adolescent development

A Model of Engaging the Family: Charla de Lupus (Lupus Chat)® Program

Charla de Lupus (Lupus Chat)® is a unique national program offering people with lupus and their families peer health support and education since 1994. Serving everyone impacted by lupus, the program seeks to reach Latinos/Hispanics and African Americans with lupus and their families. As a bilingual, bicultural program Charla intervenes with patients on multiple levels: individually, through in-person support at partner rheumatology clinics; at the community level, through participation in community health fairs and hosting special events; and on a group level, through support groups [8].

One of the core components of their program is their Teen, Young Adult, and Parent Support Group. This psychoeducational group invites guest speakers, such as rheumatologists or other allied health professionals, to provide educational opportunities for the entire family to learn about lupus, discuss topics to enhance family relationships, and better cope with lupus. The program is staffed by a clinical social worker and a peer health educator who work collaboratively to meet the needs of the whole family and address the individual needs of either the parent or patient impacted by lupus. Clinical staff also support families through increasing their knowledge about lupus, promoting health-directed behaviors, supporting effective coping strategies, and enhancing access to care and community resources. The group also offers breakout sessions for both the teens and parents where they have a safe space to exchange stories with peers and learn new coping techniques, strategies, and resources.

The program has evaluated its impact in reaching diverse communities through their family model of support. Program evaluation underscored the relevance of the family model of support when serving chronically ill diverse teens and young adults with SLE and their caregivers. Community programs like Charla are an important resource for rheumatology providers—given effective engagement of the family and support system in caring for the whole patient [9].

References

1. Bokhari SFH, Mushtaq A. Psychosocial aspects of rheumatic disease management: addressing mental health and well-being. Cureus. 2023;15(11):e49267.
2. Golics CJ, Basra MKA, Finlay AY, Salek S. The impact of disease on family members: a critical aspect of medical care. J R Soc Med. 2013;106(10):399–407.
3. Bennett WL, Pitts S, Aboumatar H, Sharma R, Smith BM, Das A et al. Strategies for patient, family, and caregiver engagement. 2020.
4. Siminoff LA. Incorporating patient and family preferences into evidence-based medicine. BMC Med Inform Decis Mak. 2013;13(Suppl 3):S6.
5. The American Academy of Child and Adolescent Psychiatry. Adolescent Development Part II. 2017. Available from: https://www.aacap.org/AACAP/Families_and_Youth/Facts_for_Families/FFF-Guide/Normal-Adolescent-Development-Part-II-058.aspx

6. Knight A, Vickery M, Fiks AG, Barg FK. The illness experience of youth with lupus/mixed connective tissue disease: a mixed methods analysis of patient and parent perspectives. Lupus. 2016;25(9):1028–39.
7. Tunnicliffe DJ, Singh-Grewal D, Chaitow J, Mackie F, Manolios N, Lin MW, et al. Lupus means sacrifices: perspectives of adolescents and young adults with systemic lupus erythematosus. Arthritis Care Res. 2016;68(6):828–37.
8. Hospital for Special Surgery. Charla de Lupus (Lupus Chat)®. 2024. Available from: https://www.hss.edu/charladelupus.asp
9. Flores MT, Rose JA, Toral P, Horton R, Pichardo DM, Mendez L, et al. Evaluating the Charla De Lupus (Lupus Chat)(R) program's teen, young adult and parent support group: reaching the Hispanic/Latino community through a family model of support. In: Arthritis & rheumatology. Hoboken: Wiley; 2016.

10 Self-Management and Patient Education Interventions

According to the CDC, "an estimated 54 million Americans are currently living with a rheumatic disease" [1]. Research has widely supported the role of self-management and patient education interventions to help people manage chronic conditions, reducing patient symptoms and improving overall quality of life. The goals of self-management are to help patients learn new and realistic strategies they can implement in their daily life to help them make informed decisions about managing their condition. For example, learning how to set goals or track your symptoms is an important self-management skill. Additionally, self-management can: improve the patient's self-confidence and skills in managing physical and emotional symptoms associated with the rheumatic condition; support doctor-patient communication; and promote new health-directed behaviors or lifestyle changes [2, 3].

Several other studies have demonstrated the value of self-management interventions in managing rheumatic conditions:

- A study that looked at the effectiveness of self-management interventions in inflammatory arthritis (IA) highlights the importance of incorporating self-management interventions in routine clinical care and the need for additional research on IA with a focus on which intervention components contribute most to achieving better critical outcomes. It also highlights

J. Rose-Smith et al., *The Psychosocial Impact of Rheumatic Conditions*, https://doi.org/10.1007/978-3-031-95338-5_10

the many benefits of different components of self-management, including disease specific education, problem-solving, goal-setting, patient education, cognitive behavioral therapy, and more [4].

- A study looking at the use of self-management strategies for people with persistent musculoskeletal disorders reports that self-management strategies are essential to the management of persistent musculoskeletal disorders, while also highlighting the role of physical therapists. They describe the components of what "good" self-management support should address. According to findings, in order to facilitate effective self-management, one should (1) help the patient to identify his or her barriers and goals, (2) assist in identifying optimal strategies to reduce or avoid symptom exacerbation through problem-solving, and (3) support the patient in identifying ways to measure the effectiveness of self-management [5].
- Another study that aimed to identify the support needs of outpatients with rheumatic disorders found that patients viewed self-management as their own process. However, they also found benefit in support from professionals and loved ones. When working with professionals, self-management support should focus on coaching patients in problem-solving skills to manage the medical, emotional, and social challenges of living with a rheumatic condition [6].

Self-Efficacy and Self-Management

As discussed, living with a rheumatic condition can profoundly impact all areas of a person's life. Studies reinforce the value of self-management programs and disease-specific patient education interventions in improving overall self-management skills in managing chronic conditions. Further factors that can impact strong self-management include patients with multiple rheumatic conditions, language barriers, and how individuals cope with their condition. These factors can impact whether an individual will have strong or poor self-management of their condition and other health-related outcomes. Self-efficacy refers to an individual's belief or confidence in their ability to manage certain behaviors. Research reinforces that high self-efficacy is an important predictor of an individual's ability to manage their chronic disease symptoms. Patients with higher self-efficacy have a stronger sense of control in managing challenges associated with living with a chronic condition [7, 8].

Dr. Kate Lorig is known for her work on chronic disease and patient education. Her research has focused on the development and evaluation of self-management programs in English and Spanish for people with chronic diseases. Her research at Stanford University included the creation of the Arthritis Self-Management Program, which demonstrated that small group peer-led arthritis programs could impact health status and health behaviors. Based on this research, the US National Arthritis Foundation disseminated this program nationally [9].

Given the important correlation between self-efficacy to manage chronic disease and health-related quality of life, measuring a person's self-efficacy through a self-reported questionnaire can be a highly valuable tool for providers caring for patients with rheumatic disease. The Self-Efficacy for Managing Chronic Disease Scale is a 6-item scale developed to measure changes in self-efficacy in program participants and has been used in numerous evaluations of chronic disease self-management programs across several chronic conditions, including arthritis, diabetes, and cancer [10, 11].

Health Literacy and Self-Management

Healthy People 2030 defines and addresses both personal health literacy and organizational health literacy, as follows [12]:

- **Personal health literacy** is the degree to which individuals have the ability to find, understand, and use information and services to inform health-related decisions and actions for themselves and others.

- **Organizational health literacy** is the degree to which organizations equitably enable individuals to find, understand, and use information and services to inform health-related decisions and actions for themselves and others [13].

About "36 percent of adults in the U.S. have low health literacy" [14]. Populations at risk for low health literacy experience multiple health disparities, including access to care, ineffective communication with healthcare providers, and decreased treatment adherence. Individuals with high literacy skills may still experience challenges with low health literacy skills in specific situations. This is especially relevant in patients with rheumatic conditions, who are faced with physical and emotional stressors that can impact how patients access health information and their ability to follow up with treatment recommendations.

Health literacy is more than the ability to read and understand specific information. It includes being able to act on the information provided, such as understanding how to properly take and dose medication or following instructions before a procedure. Other barriers may impact communication, especially when there are differences in culture, gender, sexual orientation, race, socioeconomic status, religion, age, and language between provider and patient. Low health literacy is associated with a greater risk of poorer overall health outcomes, including recurrent visits to the emergency room, more hospital stays, poor medication compliance, and a lack of routine follow-up care for disease management. Patients with higher health literacy skills can be more involved and active partners in healthcare decision-making [15, 16].

As providers, it's essential to be aware of the impact that health literacy has on the overall health outcomes of the often diverse communities impacted by rheumatic conditions at higher rates.

Below are some tips for providers as well as communication and health literacy tools for providers to use in their practice or when developing patient education interventions.

Tips for Providers to Promote Health Literacy

- Assess your own verbal and nonverbal communication so you are more aware of how you communicate.
- Demonstrate interest, curiosity, understanding, and empathy when communicating with patients to reduce uncertainty and enhance patient confidence.
- Use health literacy screenings to assess the populations you serve.
- Schedule interpreter services in advance of appointments when working with patients with limited English proficiency patients.
- Refer patients to disease-specific support and education programs or other resources [17].

Communication and Health Literacy Tools for Providers

Ask-Tell-Ask is an interactive tool that asks the patient about their beliefs and values and how they would like to receive information to facilitate shared decision-making. It emphasizes the provider's role as an interactive guide rather than a one-way supplier of information. This strategy can help patients and providers efficiently negotiate important healthcare decisions. Here is an example of how a provider might implement this tool.

Ask the patient to describe their preferences for learning and their understanding of the issue, diagnosis, medication, treatment plan, etc.:

- *How do you like information given to you, in clinical or lay terms?*
- *How do you understand your disease/medication/treatment?*

Tell the patient what they need to know in plain, simple-to-understand language:

- Use short, easy-to-understand statements, and avoid medical jargon.

Ask the patient to tell you what they understood or what their decision is [18, 19].

Ask Me 3® is a tool developed by health literacy experts that encourages patients to ask three simple questions each time they talk to a care team member. It is designed to improve communication between patients and their providers. The technique encourages patients to ask three important questions during every medical visit. It can be helpful for providers to educate their patients on these questions [20, 21], as it supports them in being more active members of their healthcare:

1. **What is my main problem?**
2. **What do I need to do?**
3. **Why is it important for me to do this?**

Single Item Literacy Screener (SILS) is an evidence-based tool with one question that helps to identify adult patients with limited reading ability who need help reading health-related materials. The SILS was created to specifically assess adult literacy in medicine and is scored on a scale from 1 to 5, where 1 = never and 5 = always. The question is: *How often do you need to have someone help you when you read instructions, pamphlets, or other written material from your doctor or pharmacy?* [22, 23].

Support and Education Programs: Why Do They Matter?

Patient education interventions, such as support groups, psychoeducational workshops, and peer counseling, have been shown to improve health outcomes, self-efficacy, and satisfaction with treatment among patients with different chronic conditions. These interventions can reduce isolation associated with living with a chronic disease, address psychosocial barriers, and improve patient compliance with treatment. Additionally, patient interventions support those living with a chronic condition to take an active role in their care, understand their condition, and connect with peers who can share strategies for coping with physical and emotional challenges.

Research reinforces the efficacy of targeted approaches to patient education interventions: "A 2016 multidisciplinary European League Against Rheumatism (EULAR) task force included evidence-based recommendations for incorporating patient education as an integral component of standard care for people with inflammatory arthritis" [24]. In addition, a study looking at peer counseling/health education interventions in lupus and other rheumatology illnesses reported improved outcomes for self-efficacy, mental health status, and fatigue [25].

A Specialty Hospital Example: National Support and Education Programs

A rheumatology and orthopedic specialty hospital provides disease-specific national support and education programs for SLE, rheumatoid arthritis, and myositis. Their evidenced-based programs conduct needs assessments based on patient feedback to determine their program's impact, satisfaction, and reach. These programs are culturally tailored, offered in multiple languages, and are developmentally specific. Their psychoeducational support groups include lectures by rheumatology and multidisciplinary experts to provide education and create a space for group discussions. All of these programs are facilitated by professional social workers and program associates/peers who themselves are living with the condition.[1]

(continued)

[1] https://www.hss.edu/social-work-programs.asp. Last visited: 04-28-2023

Several studies conducted at this specialty hospital reinforce the benefit of patient education interventions in the management of lupus and rheumatoid arthritis:

- A study evaluating a psychoeducational program found that a support group addressed the psychological and educational needs of people with lupus with notable increases in the impact of four core areas: knowledge, coping, self-management, and social support [26].
- Another study looking at a support and education group for newly diagnosed patients with rheumatoid arthritis (RA) found a positive effect on group members' ability to make more informed decisions regarding their RA, improved coping, and communication with their providers and more hope about their condition [27].

Best Practice Examples for Lupus Programs Interventions

LupusLine® Program is a free telephone counseling service that provides one-to-one support for people with lupus. It is the only national, hospital-based telephone peer support program that links people who are referred to the service with trained volunteers who have lupus—whether living in the New York tristate region, across the country, or internationally. Following a talk with a professional social worker, callers are individually matched with a trained volunteer who shares a special understanding of living with lupus. The program completes a psychosocial assessment of its callers to closely match patients with particular concerns with counselors who may have had those same medical or social life experiences. The program supports patients living with lupus in the following ways:

- Assists with adjustment to a new diagnosis.
- Improves communication with family and medical providers.

- Identifies new coping strategies.
- Enhances understanding of diagnosis and symptoms to improve self-efficacy.
- Provides emotional support.

In over the 30 years of its existence, the program has been evaluated several times to understand the impact on the callers utilizing the service as well as the impact on the volunteers who themselves provide the support and education interventions. Studies reinforced that the LupusLine® model offers substantial benefit to people coping with the complex, ongoing psychosocial challenges of SLE. Users of the service identified less depression, anxiety, and isolation as a result of their involvement in the program [28, 29].

References

1. American College of Rheumatology. New ACR White Paper Highlights Health Care Challenges Affecting the Rheumatic Disease Community: American College of Rheumatology. 2021. https://rheumatology.org/press-releases/new-acr-white-paper-highlights-health-care-challenges-affecting-the-rheumatic-disease-community. Accessed 28 Apr 2021.
2. What Is Self-Management Education?: Centers for Disease Control and Prevention, National Center for Chronic Disease Prevention and Health Promotion, Division of Population Health. 2018. cdc.gov/learnmorefeelbetter/sme/index.htm. Accessed 28 Apr 2021.
3. Anekwe TD, Rahkovsky I. Self-management: a comprehensive approach to management of chronic conditions. Am J Public Health. 2018;108(S6):S430–S6.
4. Marques A, Santos E, Nikiphorou E, Bosworth A, Carmona L. Effectiveness of self-management interventions in inflammatory arthritis: a systematic review informing the 2021 EULAR recommendations for the implementation of self-management strategies in patients with inflammatory arthritis. RMD Open. 2021;7(2):e001647.
5. Hutting N, Johnston V, Staal JB, Heerkens YF. Promoting the use of self-management strategies for people with persistent musculoskeletal disorders: the role of physical therapists. J Orthop Sports Phys Ther. 2019;49(4):212–5.
6. Been-Dahmen JM, Walter MJ, Dwarswaard J, Hazes JM, van Staa A, Ista E. What support is needed to self-manage a rheumatic disorder: a qualitative study. BMC Musculoskelet Disord. 2017;18(1):84.

7. Chan SW. Chronic disease management, self-efficacy and quality of life. J Nurs Res. 2021;29(1):e129.
8. Dishman RK, Motl RW, Sallis JF, Dunn AL, Birnbaum AS, Welk GJ, et al. Self-management strategies mediate self-efficacy and physical activity. Am J Prev Med. 2005;29(1):10–8.
9. CDC. Self-Management Education Workshops: Centers for Disease Control and Prevention, National Center for Chronic Disease Prevention and Health Promotion, Division of Population Health. 2020. https://www.cdc.gov/arthritis/interventions/self_manage.htm. Accessed 28 Apr 2021.
10. Self-Efficacy for Managing Chronic Disease 6-item Scale: Self Management Resource Center. https://selfmanagementresource.com/wp-content/uploads/English_-_self-efficacy_for_managing_chronic_disease_6-item.pdf. Accessed 28 Apr 2021.
11. Ritter PL, Lorig K. The English and Spanish self-efficacy to manage chronic disease scale measures were validated using multiple studies. J Clin Epidemiol. 2014;67(11):1265–73.
12. U.S. Department of Health and Human Services. Health Literacy in Healthy People 2030: Office of Disease Prevention and Health Promotion, Office of the Assistant Secretary for Health, Office of the Secretary, U.S. Department of Health and Human Services. https://health.gov/healthypeople/priority-areas/health-literacy-healthy-people-2030. Accessed 28 Apr 2021.
13. CDC. Health Literacy: Centers for Disease Control and Prevention. 2023. https://www.cdc.gov/healthliteracy/learn/index.html. Accessed 28 Apr 2021.
14. Health Literacy Fact Sheets: Center for Health Care Strategies. 2013. https://www.chcs.org/resource/health-literacy-fact-sheets/. Accessed 28 Apr 2021.
15. An Introduction to Health Literacy: National Library of Medicine. https://www.nnlm.gov/guides/intro-shealth-literacy. Accessed 28 Apr 2021.
16. van der Gaag M, Heijmans M, Spoiala C, Rademakers J. The importance of health literacy for self-management: a scoping review of reviews. Chronic Illn. 2022;18(2):234–54.
17. National Health Initiatives: Resources for Implementation: Office of Disease Prevention and Health Promotion. 2022. https://health.gov/our-work/national-health-initiatives/health-literacy/health-literate-care-model/resources-implementation. Accessed 28 Apr 2021.
18. What Is "Ask, Tell, Ask"?: Institute for Healthcare Improvement. 2016. https://www.ihi.org/education/IHIOpenSchool/resources/Pages/AudioandVideo/ConnieDavis-WhatIsAskTellAsk.aspx. Accessed 28 Apr 2021.
19. Gaster B, Edwards K, Trinidad SB, Gallagher TH, Braddock CH 3rd. Patient-centered discussions about prostate cancer screening: a real-world approach. Ann Intern Med. 2010;153(10):661–5.

20. Ask Me 3: Good Questions for Your Good Health: Institute for Healthcare Improvement. https://www.ihi.org/resources/Pages/Tools/Ask-Me-3-Good-Questions-for-Your-Good-Health.aspx. Accessed 28 Apr 2021.
21. Lord J, Borkowski N, Weech-Maldonado R. Patient engagement in home health: the role of health literacy and "Ask me three®". Home Health Care Manag Pract. 2021;33(3):202–9.
22. Bonaccorsi G, Grazzini M, Pieri L, Santomauro F, Ciancio M, Lorini C. Assessment of health literacy and validation of single-item literacy screener (SILS) in a sample of Italian people. Ann Ist Super Sanita. 2017;53(3):205–12.
23. Morris NS, MacLean CD, Chew LD, Littenberg B. The single item literacy screener: evaluation of a brief instrument to identify limited reading ability. BMC Fam Pract. 2006;7:21.
24. Combe B, Landewe R, Daien CI, Hua C, Aletaha D, Álvaro-Gracia JM, et al. 2016 update of the EULAR recommendations for the management of early arthritis. Ann Rheum Dis. 2017;76(6):948–59.
25. Williams EM, Penfield M, Kamen D, Oates JC. An intervention to reduce psychosocial and biological indicators of stress in African American lupus patients: the balancing lupus experiences with stress strategies study. Open J Prev Med. 2014;4(1):22–31.
26. Flores MT, Horton R, Rose JA, Paget SA, Lockshin M. The SLE workshop: an evaluation of a long-standing hospital-based psychoeducational program. In: Arthritis & rheumatology. Hoboken: Wiley-Blackwell; 2015.
27. EurekAlert. Study shows rheumatoid arthritis support and education program has strong positive impact: EurekAlert. 2014. https://www.eurekalert.org/news-releases/742804. Accessed 28 Apr 2021.
28. Toral P, Flores MT, Horton R, Rose J. Evaluation of a longstanding telephone peer counseling service on people with systemic lupus erythematosus and their loved ones. In: Arthritis & rheumatology. Hoboken: Wiley; 2017.
29. Horton R, Peterson MGE, Powell S, Engelhard E, Paget SA. Users evaluate lupusline a telephone peer counseling service. Arthritis Rheum. 1997;10(4):257–63.

11 Health Disparities and Confronting Implicit Bias as a Strategy to Address Them

What Are Health Disparities?

Health disparities continue to be key drivers of premature death and deepening adverse healthcare outcomes, especially for racially and ethnically diverse populations, women, the uninsured and underinsured, and those impacted by poverty. Healthy People 2030 defines a health disparity as "a particular type of health difference that is closely linked with social, economic, and/or environmental disadvantage. Health disparities adversely affect groups of people who have systematically experienced greater obstacles to health based on their: racial or ethnic group; religion; socioeconomic status; gender; age; mental health; cognitive, sensory, or physical disability; sexual orientation or gender identity; geographic location; or other characteristics historically linked to discrimination or exclusion" [1].

Health disparities in rheumatology are well-documented, especially for common rheumatic conditions such as SLE and RA. Several studies have demonstrated the continued impact of health disparities on different populations with rheumatic illness based on race, ethnicity, and socioeconomic and insurance status, including the following:

- Research shows that Hispanic RA patients experience delays in receiving care despite being younger and having greater disease severity [2].

J. Rose-Smith et al., *The Psychosocial Impact of Rheumatic Conditions*, https://doi.org/10.1007/978-3-031-95338-5_11

- Non-Hispanic minority patients with psoriasis in the US report fewer ambulatory visits and are less likely to have visited a dermatologist [3].
- Lower socioeconomic status is associated with worse functional status in a US cohort of RA patients [4].
- A significant portion of lupus nephritis patients on Medicaid have poor access to healthcare and do not receive appropriate therapy [5].
- Black RA patients are more likely to receive prednisone and conventional Disease-Modifying Antirheumatic Drugs (DMARDs), and less likely to receive biologics [6].
- Hurried provider communication was associated with findings on the damage index of the Systemic Lupus Erythematosus International Collaborating Clinics (SLICC), showing damage accrual in African American SLE patients [7].

Drivers of Health Disparities

There are many different drivers of health disparities in rheumatology, both within and outside of medical care (Fig. 11.1).

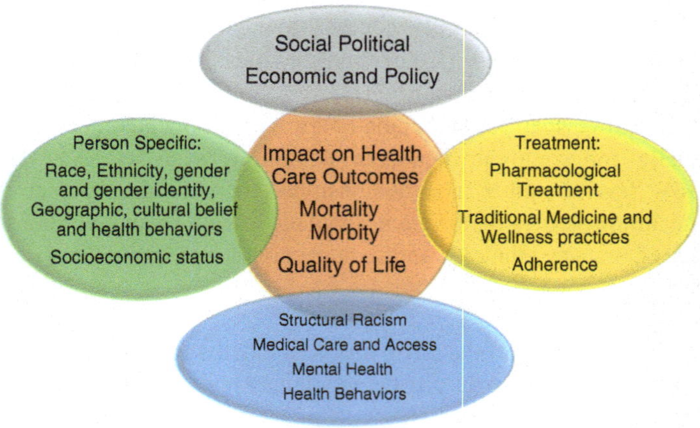

Fig. 11.1 Drivers of health disparities

Non-medical Drivers of Health

According to Healthy People 2030, social determinants of health (SDOH) are the conditions in the environments where people are born, live, learn, work, play, worship, and age that affect a wide range of health, functioning, and quality-of-life outcomes and risks [8]. One's social environment can significantly impact health outcomes. Chap. 12 dives deeper into SDOH and health-related social needs and offers examples of strategies that can be implemented on both a provider and system level to address these issues (Fig. 11.2).

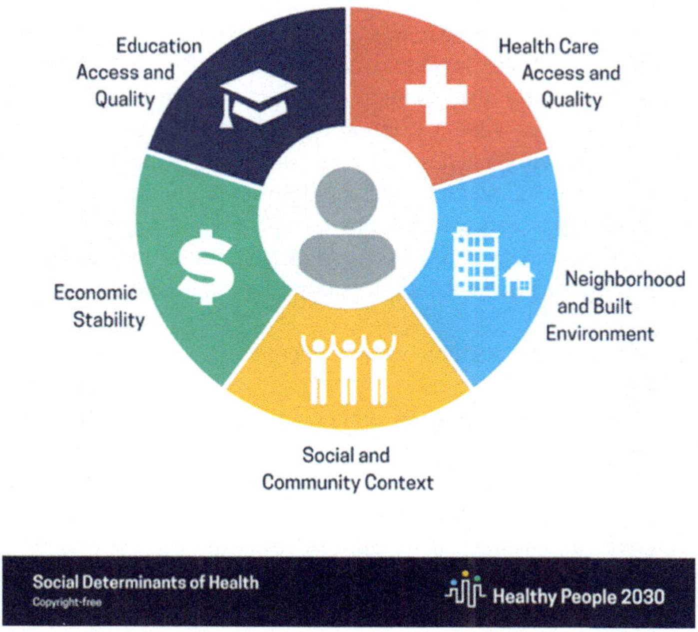

Fig. 11.2 Social determinants of health wheel. (Source [1])

Confronting Implicit Bias: A Strategy Clinicians Can Use to Address Health Disparities

Examining our own biases as clinicians, what we bring to the table, and understanding how to debias our actions has proven to be an important first step in addressing disparities.

Implicit Bias

Implicit bias refers to the attitudes and stereotypes that affect our understanding, actions, and decisions in an unconscious manner. The implicit associations we have in our unconscious can cause us to have feelings about others based on characteristics such as language, gender, appearance, race, ethnicity, age, and class [9]. These associations develop over the course of a lifetime, beginning at an early age through exposure to direct and indirect messages about what we are supposed to think and feel [10]. These associations can subtly affect how we, as healthcare providers, perceive, interact with, and deliver care to our patients.

Stereotypes and assumptions can perpetuate negative biases that can put others at risk for harm or isolation or prevent people from accessing needed care. It is important to be mindful of:

- Our language and how we label people.
- Stereotypical "jokes".
- The way we treat each other and the diverse communities we serve.

Anyone can get sick, regardless of race or ethnicity, and one way we can ensure that we are providing the highest quality of care for all people is by becoming more aware of our own biases and taking action to address them.

Why Is Understanding Implicit Bias Important?

Two landmark reports by the Institute of Medicine, *Crossing the Quality Chasm* (2001) and *Unequal Treatment* (2002), highlighted pervasive racial and ethnic disparities in the US healthcare system [11, 12]. The reports found that even when they had the same insurance and socioeconomic status as nonminorities—and when comorbidities, stage of presentation, and other confounders were controlled for—minorities often received lower-quality healthcare.

Research shows that part of what causes disparities are the implicit biases of healthcare workers, which can unintentionally lead to providing lower-quality care for patients. The literature shows that implicit bias based on race, gender, sexual orientation, weight, insurance, and other group identification can affect providers':

- Quality of clinical encounter.
- Diagnostic decision-making.
- Symptom management.
- Treatment recommendations.
- Referrals to specialty care.
- Interpersonal behaviors, such as communication, empathy, and trust [13]

Reports indicate that the coronavirus does not discriminate; however, people who are disproportionately affected by health disparities and poor social determinants of health—such as low access to healthcare, poverty, housing, and food insecurity—with consequent higher comorbidities, have significantly higher risk of being affected by COVID-19 with worse health outcomes.

What Factors Put Us at Risk for Implicit Bias?

Research shows that various factors can put us at risk for implicit bias. These include the following:

- Emotional states such as anger, anxiety, fear, and disgust.
- Lack of concrete guidelines for decision-making.
- Being distracted or pressured.
- Long hours.
- Working in a fast-paced work environment.
- Dealing with crises.
- Being backlogged.
- Lack of feedback [14]

Therefore, it is important that we are aware of the unintended biases that can affect our work with patients and how to address them.

Starting Where the Client Is

> People fail to get along because they fear each other; they fear each other because they don't know each other; they don't know each other because they have not communicated with each other.
> –Martin Luther King Jr

Cultural norms and beliefs, stereotypes, stigma, and implicit bias often mediate the doctor-patient encounter. Both patients and providers can bring factors such as stress, mistrust, time pressures, and poor communication to the doctor-patient encounter that can lead to biased treatment decisions, poor adherence, and, ultimately, negative outcomes.

Implicit bias has been described by Banaji and Greenwald as our "blind spot" [15]. Being aware of what we bring to our interactions with patients and being intentional about how we engage patients to build trusting relationships are key to avoiding those blind spots. We are the most important tool in our interactions with patients. It is important that we start where the client is and practice from a patient-centered care model. This often allows the clinician to see and consider the whole person versus negatively labeling the patient or making assumptions.

What Can I Do to Address Implicit Bias?

Addressing implicit bias is not always easy; it is a process. However, as clinicians, we are often seen as having the power and influence over decision-making for patients, and there are steps we can take to learn how to identify and address unconscious thoughts that can unintentionally influence patient care.

Make a Personal Commitment to Learn More About Your Implicit Biases

- You can start by taking the implicit association test (IAT) to help identify any hidden biases.
- Take the time to reflect on your results. Remember, the IAT shows that:
  - Implicit biases are pervasive, and everyone possesses them.
  - We generally tend to hold implicit biases that favor the groups we identify with.
  - Implicit biases are flexible. The implicit associations we have formed can be gradually unlearned through various "de-biasing" techniques.
  - Using what you have learned, work on developing an understanding of the potential for unconscious bias in your work, and make a commitment to be alert.

Practice from a Stance of Dignity and Respect

- Seek to learn about diverse cultural and health beliefs.
- Cultivating awareness and sensitivity can be more effective in acknowledging differences in diversity [16].
- Make an effort to be inclusive—everyone is valued, and all contributions are welcome.
  - For example, respect the gender identity of patients by using their self-identified names and pronouns in your interactions with them.

- Do not support jokes that disrespect any group of people.
- View people as individuals instead of as part of a larger group.
- Practice patient-centered care—build partnerships with patients and their support person(s).
- View yourself as part of a larger group to increase empathy and trust.

Be Conscious of Your Decision-Making Process and Check for Bias

- Use established guidelines, assessments, checklists, or process flows for doing your work, as appropriate.
- Avoid making assumptions/judgments based on first glance or "eyeballing" patients.
- Document the reasoning behind your decisions.
- Use shared decision-making tools to allow for enhanced communication, education, and patient input related to the care plan.

Identify Sources of Stress and Factors That Contribute to Pressure in the Environment

- Work to minimize stressful situations that can cause you to rely on automatic thinking and lead to biased decisions.
- Practice mindfulness: Take a few moments between cases, meetings, etc., to clear your mind and refocus on the next task.

Develop a Spirit of Curiosity

- Get to know your patients beyond their diagnosis:
  - Assess for social determinants of health.
    - Ask patients about their social history to better support and understand the challenges they face.

  - Not assessing social history or challenges can lead to an inappropriate care plan.
  - For example, the patient may not be able to afford prescribed medication.
  - Practice selective inquiry based on clinical considerations.
  - Look for "clinical red flags."
  - For example, child abuse/elder abuse/domestic violence.
- Use the teach-back method and Ask Me 3® techniques to enhance communication and improve outcomes between the provider and client [17, 18].
- Utilize motivational interviewing techniques when assessing patients to focus on having an open dialogue to explore a patient's readiness for change rather than traditional advice-giving. This helps to identify barriers to change and decrease resistance.
- Other strategies to combat implicit bias include:
  - Stereotype replacement: Recognizing that a response is based on a stereotype and consciously adjusting the response.
  - Counter-stereotypic imaging: Imagining the individual as the opposite of the stereotype.
  - Individuation: Seeing the person as an individual rather than a stereotype (e.g., learning about their personal history and the context that brought them to the doctor's office or health center).
  - Perspective taking: "Putting yourself in the other person's shoes".
  - Increasing opportunities for contact with individuals from different groups: Expanding one's network of friends and colleagues or attending events where people of other racial and ethnic groups, gender identities, sexual orientations, and other groups may be present.
  - Partnership building: Reframing the interaction with the patient as one between collaborating equals rather than between a high-status person and a low-status person.

– Utilizing the teach-back method: As previously discussed, teach-back is a method that can be used to confirm the patient's understanding of healthcare instructions and is associated with improved adherence, quality, and patient safety.

References

1. Health Equity in Healthy People 2030. Available from: https://health.gov/healthypeople/priority-areas/health-equity-healthy-people-2030
2. Riad M, Dunham DP, Chua JR, Shakoor N, Hassan S, Everakes S, et al. Health disparities among Hispanics with rheumatoid arthritis: delay in presentation to rheumatologists contributes to later diagnosis and treatment. J Clin Rheumatol Pract Rep Rheum Musculoskelet Dis. 2020;26(7):279–84.
3. Fischer AH, Shin DB, Gelfand JM, Takeshita J. Health care utilization for psoriasis in the United States differs by race: an analysis of the 2001-2013 medical expenditure panel surveys. J Am Acad Dermatol. 2018;78(1):200–3.
4. Li J, Schmajuk G, Evans M, Izadi Z, Katz P, Ogdie A, et al. Socioeconomic disparities in functional status among RA patients: a longitudinal analysis using RISE data. In: Arthritis & rheumatology. Hoboken: Wiley; 2020.
5. Yazdany J, Feldman CH, Liu J, Ward MM, Fischer MA, Costenbader KH. Quality of care for incident lupus nephritis among Medicaid beneficiaries in the United States. Arthritis Care Res. 2014;66(4):617–24. https://doi.org/10.1002/acr.22182.
6. He E, Cornblath E, Yalamanchi P, Ogdie A, Baker J, George M. Characterization of racial disparities in rheumatoid arthritis treatment choice and location of care. In: Arthritis & rheumatology. Hoboken: Wiley; 2020.
7. Sun K, Eudy AM, Criscione-Schreiber LG, Sadun RE, Rogers JL, Doss J, et al. Racial differences in patient-provider communication, patient self-efficacy, and their associations with systemic lupus erythematosus-related damage: a cross-sectional survey. J Rheumatol. 2021;48(7):1022–8.
8. Social Determinants of Health – Healthy People 2030 | health.gov [Internet]. 2024. Available from: https://health.gov/healthypeople/priority-areas/social-determinants-health
9. Capatosto K, Jackson V, Staats C, Wright R. State of the science: implicit bias review. Kirwan Institute for the Study of Race and Ethnicity, The Ohio State University; 2016. p. 3449.

10. Implicit Bias in Health Care. Quick Safety. 2016; (23).
11. Committee on Quality of Health Care in America. Crossing the quality chasm: a new health system for the 21st century. Washington: Committee on Quality of Health Care in America; 2001.
12. Smedley BD, Stith AY, Nelson AR. Unequal treatment: confronting racial and ethnic disparities in health care. Washington; 2003.
13. FitzGerald C, Hurst S. Implicit bias in healthcare professionals: a systematic review. BMC Med Ethics. 2017;18:1–18.
14. Casey PM, Warren RK, Elek JK. Helping courts address implicit bias: resources for education. National Center for State Courts; 2012.
15. Banaji MR, Greenwald AG. Blindspot: hidden biases of good people. Bantam; 2016.
16. Apfelbaum EP, Sommers SR, Norton MI. Seeing race and seeming racist? Evaluating strategic colorblindness in social interaction. J Pers Soc Psychol. 2008;95(4):918.
17. Teachbacktraining.com – Teach Back Training. 2024. Available from: https://teachbacktraining.org/
18. Ask Me 3: Good Questions for Your Good Health | Institute for Healthcare Improvement [Internet]. 2024. Available from: https://www.ihi.org/resources/tools/ask-me-3-good-questions-your-good-health

12 Beyond the Exam Room: Addressing Social Determinants of Health

Social determinants of health (SDOH) are the conditions in the environments where people work, live, and play that affect people's health, functioning, outcomes, and risks. Health-related social needs (HRSNs) are social and economic needs that people experience that affect one's ability to live a healthy life. Some of these include access to healthy food: safe and affordable housing; utilities such as heating, cooling, and clean water; safety at home; transportation to get to medical appointments and activities of daily living; social support; employment; education; and income. Research shows that 80–90% of "modifiable contributors" to healthy outcomes are SDOH: health-related behaviors, socioeconomic factors, and environmental factors [1]. Addressing SDOH, in addition to clinical interventions, can move us toward health equity for all patients.

This is important for rheumatology because someone's lived environment and access to basic needs can greatly impact their ability to follow their prescribed treatment regimen, which can improve their health outcomes.

Case Example

Mrs. Dewing was prescribed a biologic for treatment of RA. The healthcare team spent 2 months getting grants to pay for it, and this goal was finally achieved. It was a big win! However, the patient was not getting better, and her labs didn't show the drug

J. Rose-Smith et al., *The Psychosocial Impact of Rheumatic Conditions*, https://doi.org/10.1007/978-3-031-95338-5_12

in her system. Her physician became incredibly frustrated and asked the social worker to step in to see what was going on. Among the first few questions the social worker asked were, "Are you still living at XYZ address? Who lives with you?" Mrs. Dewing hung her head and said, "I lost my house a month ago and have been couch surfing and sleeping in subway cars. The medication needs to be refrigerated, and I don't have access to a refrigerator to store it." Better understanding Mrs. Dewing situation, the team implemented a plan to store the medication at the hospital, and she would come in once a week for it to be administered.

This case highlights that even the best treatment regimens can fail simply due to factors in a patient's living environment.

Many patients with rheumatic diseases see their rheumatologist as their primary care provider, sometimes seeing their rheumatologist more frequently than any other provider and establishing a strong patient-provider relationship. Given the chronic nature and complexity of the disease, rheumatologists often develop relationships with patients for extended periods of time, and thus, they are uniquely positioned to identify any SDOH needs that can critically impact a patient's treatment plan and health outcomes.

The Why: Regulatory Guidance

Accrediting and regulatory bodies are now calling for healthcare organizations to assess and address SDOH. These include Healthy People 2030, Centers for Medicare and Medicaid Services (CMS), the Joint Commission, and the US News and World Report rankings. "One of Healthy People 2030's 5 overarching goals are specifically related to SDOH: 'Create social, physical, and economic environments that promote attaining the full potential for health and well-being for all'" [2, 3].

SDOHs are an important part of national and statewide delivery systems and payment reform activities. CMS's inpatient prospective payment system (IPPS) final rule includes several health equity measures, including changes to the hospital Inpatient

Quality Reporting (IQR) program, which have a reimbursement impact (GNYHA).

The "Hospital Commitment to Health Equity" measures five domains that include: Equity as a Strategic Priority, Data Collection, Data Analysis, Quality Improvement, and Leadership Engagement. The Data Collection domain underscores that "collecting valid and reliable demographic and social determinant of health data on patients served in a hospital is an important step in identifying and eliminating health disparities." The elements include the hospital's attesting to collecting "self-reported race and ethnicity and/or social determinant of health information on the majority of our patients," "training for staff in culturally sensitive" collection of this information, and inputting this information "collected from patients into structured, interoperable data elements using certified EHR technology" [4].

Furthermore, in the Data Analysis domain, a hospital must attest to "stratifying key performance indicators by demographic and/or social determinants of health variables to identify equity gaps and include this information on hospital performance dashboards" [4, 5].

The Joint Commission Health Disparities Standard (LD.04.03.08), effective in 2023, states that "reducing health care disparities for the organizations' patients is a quality and safety priority." Aligned with committing to improving healthcare equity, hospitals must "assess the patient's health-related social needs and provide information about community resources and support services" and "identify health care disparities by stratifying quality and safety data using patient sociodemographic characteristics" [6].

Similarly, both the US News and World Report Pediatric Survey and American Hospital Association (AHA) survey include questions about screening data for SDOH and collecting this information in the electronic medical record, utilizing the data to identify health disparities in patient care/outcomes and implementing quality improvement projects designed to address these issues [7–9]. Both of these surveys feed US News and World Report rankings which are reported annually.

Implementing SDOH Screening

Because of how SDOH can impact health outcomes, it's important for rheumatology practices and hospitals to assess health-related social needs, aligned with guidance from regulatory bodies and your organization's commitment to health equity. This information can be assessed in your practice through the patient interview or through standardized screenings provided to patients through a questionnaire or directly through staff. There are several different models for collecting this information and intervening with patients.

Direct Practice Screening

As a rheumatology healthcare practitioner, you may not work in a hospital or a large organization where standardized screening for SDOH may be reasonable to implement. Or perhaps your organization is not prioritizing addressing these patient needs. Regardless of the setting in which you practice, one can integrate assessing for SDOH in a variety of ways through the patient-provider relationship.

When approaching these conversations, it's important to consider the challenges for both providers and patients. On the provider side, one may feel uncomfortable engaging in these conversations for fear of offending the patient, there may be a lack of time, or one may not feel they would be able to address these needs. On the patient side, one may feel reluctant to engage in these conversations due to stigma and shame, not wanting to be viewed or treated differently due to what they share [10]. This is exacerbated when one considers the inherent power dynamics of the patient-physician relationship and the intersections of various identities such as race, ethnicity, sex, gender identity, and ability status. Given these challenges, providers should be prepared to approach these conversations with self-awareness and sensitivity by utilizing best practice strategies.

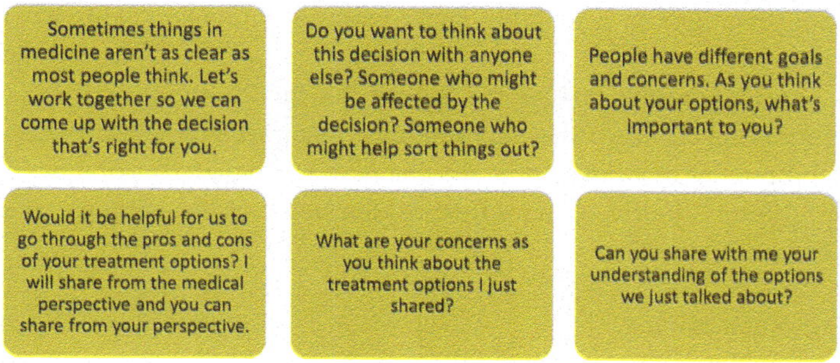

Fig. 12.1 Suggested language for healthcare providers to assess SDOH

Asking About Social History

Clinicians can ask patients about their social history to better understand and support the patient's challenges and refer them to appropriate local resources and support services. Not assessing social history and challenges can lead to inappropriate care plans—such as prescribing medication a patient cannot afford (Fig. 12.1).

Suggested Language for Asking About Social History

According to the AHA, guiding principles for SDOH screening include empathy, respect, autonomy, trust, dignity, collaboration, support, sensitivity, cultural competence, and community engagement [10]. Furthermore, Schoenthaler, Hassan, and Fiscilla discuss how adopting a relationship-centered care framework to conversations about SDOH can optimize patient engagement, comfort, and trust. Some relationship-centered strategies include adopting screenings that are family-centered, being respectful, normalizing the topic, asking permission, explaining the purpose, identifying patient strengths, expressing appreciation, and acknowledging the difficulties [11]. Key to the success of these conversations is a positive and trusting relationship with one's provider.

A natural place to discuss SDOH maybe during the social history component of the appointment. Integrating a social history component in all of your visits can help normalize this practice.

Being mindful of the principles discussed, some language one can use include:

- **Normalizing:**
  - "I ask all of my patients these questions..."
  - "We have started to ask all of our patients a few questions related to their social needs."
- **Explaining the Purpose:**
  - "I ask all my patients these questions to see if we can help address some concerns you might have so we can better care for you."
  - "I ask all my patients these questions to get a better understanding of your overall health situation."
  - "We are asking patients questions about their needs at home because we want to make sure you have access to available resources."
- **Asking Permission:**
  - "Would it be OK for us to talk about how things are going for you and your family at home?"
  - "Can I ask you a few questions about your needs at home?"

Some examples of questions to integrate with the patient visit about specific social needs:

- **Mental Health:**
  - "Last time you shared with me that you were feeling sad. Can you tell me a little more about that? Has feeling sad caused you to miss taking your medications?"
- **Social Support:**
  - "I know you live alone and you are trying to manage your healthcare in the best way. You have reported feeling more fatigued lately."

- "Is there anyone who can call us if there is an emergency?"
- "Is there anyone who helps you cook or take care of grocery shopping and cleaning?"

- **Transportation/Financial:**
  - "I noticed you missed a few appointments in the past three months and have been late for all of the appointments that you are able to make."
  - "Has something changed for you lately?"
  - "What are the barriers to you making your appointment?"
  - "I know you live 45 mins from here—how do you usually get here?"
  - "Who takes care of your children while you are at work or at your appointment?"

Standardized Organization-Wide Collection

Assembling the Interdisciplinary Workgroup

In order to successfully implement SDOH screening in a standardized way, it's critical to have key stakeholder support, especially from senior leadership invested in this initiative. Once your organization or practice decides that they would like to move forward with asking for this information, you want to ensure that you have the appropriate team members at the table across departments. Some important key players are representatives/leadership from various departments, including: population health/health equity; quality and values; nursing leadership; nurse education; physician champions; information technology; legal/compliance; and health information management. This team can formulate a workgroup that meets regularly to plan the strategy and project plan with timelines for rolling out SDOH screening.

Some key decisions need to be made to appropriately plan for collection and intervention. Your workgroup needs to decide what level of screening and intervention will take place. Does your workgroup want to start with collecting the information only to meet regulatory requirements? Or is your organization committing to both collecting the information and intervening/

addressing the HRSNs identified? Your organization or practice decisions in these areas will impact the level of effort and resources required to implement SDOH. For some, it may not be realistic to go "all in" with collection, intervention, and follow-up due to a lack of resources and time. So it's important to determine which model your organization is capable of implementing with key stakeholders—with a focus on what is best for patient care and the patient experience.

Identifying the Screening Tool

Next, the team will need to make decisions on what the screening tool will look like. This includes deciding which HRSNs should be included in the screening, which options should be considered a positive screen, and how positive screens will be operationalized. According to the CMS requirements, which specifically ask about patients 18+ years old who have an inpatient stay, the HRSN categories include food insecurity, housing stability, utilities, transportation, and safety [4]. The US News and World Report Pediatric Survey and AHA surveys include questions about education/health literacy, income/financial strain, and employment. Furthermore, the AHA Survey asks about social isolation and health behaviors.

At this time, the requirements do not dictate the specific questions to be asked. There are several existing tools to assess this information—some of these include the PRAPARE tool[1] and the Accountable Health Communities Health-Related Social Needs Screening Tool from CMS [12]. For additional options to consider, a comparison chart is available via University of California, San Francisco (UCSF), which has categorized tools by those for adult/all populations and those specifically designed for pediatric populations [13]. Your questions should also include the option to decline or indicate if the information was unable to be obtained due to the patient's condition.

In addition to choosing the questions themselves, the workgroup must define the elements of each question that trigger a

[1] https://prapare.org/the-prapare-screening-tool/. Last visited: 04-21-2023

"positive screen." For example, if you are using the Hunger Vital Sign™ Tool [14, 15], a 2-item questionnaire that has been validated to screen for food insecurity, it's important to know the tool identifies households as being at risk for food insecurity if they answer that either or both of the questions are "often true" or "sometimes true," as opposed to "never true."

If your organization is planning to not only collect but also intervene, your workgroup must also decide whether or not to include questions to [1] assess if the patient wants help and [2] indicate whether or not this is an urgent or emergent situation.

Workflow Design for Collection

Once the tool has been solidified, the workgroup should work on designing the workflow for how this information should be captured and at what point patients should interface with the screening. A process map is particularly useful to make this clear, which can also be used by your IT team to create the build needed. Some important questions include the following:

- In what format will patients be prompted by these questions? Will this take the form of a questionnaire to be completed by the patient in advance of their appointment? Or will these questions be asked verbally by staff?
- Should the questions be provided to patients via a paper survey or documented electronically through their patient portal?
- Who will be responsible for collecting the information?
- Who will be reviewing completed screenings for positive screenings?
- How often do you want to ask patients these questions? Is a one-time ask enough, or should this be done every visit, every 6 months, or annually?

Some healthcare organizations may want to begin by piloting their question to get feedback to inform the next phase of screening. This can be done utilizing a paper survey distributed by nurses during the rooming process or provided to patients by registration (or other staff) in the waiting room.

If your healthcare organization is looking to screen as many patients as possible, it would be crucial to build the screener into the EHR used by your organization so that this information can be more easily tracked, monitored, and reported on. Depending on the model your workgroup chooses (collection only vs. collection plus intervention), one can build SDOH questions into the patient portal for patients to fill out themselves electronically in advance of their appointment. Or, your workgroup may decide that in addition to patients answering these questions, staff such as nurses or social workers should review this information with patients during their appointment or ask the questions if they have not previously answered these questions.

Pros of providing the opportunity to share this information in advance include allowing patients to respond nonverbally and privately, which may lead to more honest feedback. Additionally, this saves staff time when the patient comes in for their appointment because nurses/clinical staff will not need to ask all questions but instead confirm the answers or see if any responses have changed. However, it's important to keep in mind that it depends—as some patients may feel more comfortable sharing this information with clinical staff, especially when approaching the topic in the context of a positive patient-provider relationship.

It will also be important to consider how the questions are presented to patients, so they understand the purpose of asking the questions. If presenting the questions in the patient portal, some introductory language sharing why the questions are being asked can help address patient concerns about filling out the information. Since the questions can be interpreted as sensitive, patients may initially be hesitant to complete the questionnaire without knowing how the information will be used. Similarly, if the questions are being asked by clinical staff, introductory scripting explaining the purpose should be used to facilitate understanding.

Workflow Design for Intervention

When implementing a "collection plus intervention" type of SDOH model, the workgroup should create the workflow outlining what the intervention will look like for patients who screen positive. Some important questions include the following:

- What intervention, if any, will take place when a patient screens positive for each HRSN?
- Is the same intervention expected for each positive screen?
- Will some questions trigger a more urgent intervention than others?

There are several different models for intervention, and the level of intervention is dependent on your organization and the resources available to commit to this rollout. Generally, once a patient has screened positive, the appropriate response would be to assist them with the needs identified. This includes navigating them to a resource either within the organization or a referral to community resources.

Due to the nature of certain domains, one may want to prompt a more urgent response depending on which domain a patient is screened for. For example, screening for food insecurity should be considered more urgent than screening for an educational need. The intervention may depend on the domain in which the patient screened positive. For less urgent needs, an intervention may be providing a list of vetted and relevant community resources to the patient. For urgent needs, the patient can be connected with a case worker or social worker. The patient can meet with them while there for their visit, or schedule a follow-up appointment. Or, if resources are available, a patient can be automatically referred to social work if they screen positive on any of the questions.

Referrals and Resources

In order to implement the intervention component successfully, a subteam should be focused on the resources and referrals component of the SDOH rollout. Here is where an organization can lean on their social work and/or case management leadership to compile resources and referrals to community-based organizations (CBOs) which are able to better meet the needs of the patients. Partnerships with CBOs can make a difference here to connect patients to the resources more seamlessly. This can also facilitate an opportunity to track whether or not the patient connects to the CBO and identifies whether or not they are utilizing services.

When pulling together resources and referrals, it's critical to know about the population you are serving and to connect them with appropriate resources. For example, you may have patients who live locally; however, what if you have patients from out of state or another country? How will you address the needs of this population of patients? What about patients whose primary language for healthcare is not English? These are scenarios that are important to consider.

Given technological capabilities, there are features for some EHR systems that allow one to integrate a community resource directory, an external referral platform that connects people to needed resources. This can be particularly helpful for patients who are not local and need resources in other states. Some community resources directory platforms, such as UniteUs[2], support tracking and coordinating referrals so the healthcare organization can close the loop on care.

Building into the Electronic Health Record (EHR)

Once the workflows are created for collection, intervention, and follow-up, you can bring in your IT team to discuss building them into your EHR system. Their expertise will help guide how best to support the workflows developed for your healthcare team and the accessibility of this information to clinical staff to help inform patient care. Based on your workflow, key stakeholders in collaboration with IT can identify in which exact screens the questions should be located and who should be able to see this information. They can also help ensure that answers to these questions at each juncture are updated throughout the medical record, whether it's completed by a patient in their patient portal or by clinical staff. Some examples of ways to leverage IT include creating an automated message with a referral to appropriate staff (e.g., social workers) when a patient screens positive. This can help eliminate additional steps staff need to take and make the process seamless. Furthermore, a work queue could be set up for the social worker to help prioritize patients who screen positively

[2] https://uniteus.com/. Last visited: 04-21-2024

by the level of urgency. Other ways to utilize IT may be to create a way to notify providers and other members of the healthcare team when a patient screens positive and when there is an urgent need so the physician can easily consider this information for the treatment plan.

Training and Communication

Education, training, and communication with key staff will be essential to the success of your organization's SDOH rollout. Staff should generally be aware of what is meant by SDOH, how it impacts healthcare, and understand the purpose of asking these questions. Staff who are directly involved in the SDOH workflow should receive training specific to their role. For example, if clinical support staff are the primary point of collection, nurse educators can train staff on how to conduct the screening and document answers and interventions as appropriate. If social workers are involved in the intervention and referral process, they need to be aware of how they will receive referrals specifically for SDOH and what their responsibilities are to document and follow up with a patient within a given period of time. Physicians and other clinical staff should be educated on where to find this SDOH information in the EHR and be able to easily find out if a patient's needs in which they screened positively have been addressed.

Documentation and Information Sharing

As previously mentioned, documenting the screening and intervention are essential components of SDOH rollout to identify patient needs and provide appropriate interventions. The workgroup must decide which healthcare team members will be responsible for documenting SDOH and should educate and train them appropriately. In addition to this, providers are able to code social needs using the ICD-10-CM codes included in categories Z55-Z65, more commonly referred to as "Z codes" [16]· These codes refer to nonmedical factors that can contribute to patient health, such as problems with literacy and education, employment, housing, economic circumstances, social environment, primary support group, and other psychosocial concerns. These have been available since 2016; however, healthcare providers have been slow to adopt these [17].

Applying Z codes in the EHR and hospital claims can help inform treatment plans and help us better understand the SDOH needs of patient populations. Furthermore, the Office of the National Coordinator for Health Information Technology (ONC) is invested in "advancing the use of interoperable, standardized data to represent social needs and the conditions in which people live, learn, work and play" [18]; and healthcare organizations are implementing health information exchange initiatives to address SDOH issues and better coordinate care to enhance health equity.

Your organization's workgroup must work closely with IT governance, compliance, and legal teams to determine what information is appropriate to share with outside providers, being mindful of the sensitive nature of the information and safety concerns that may be identified through SDOH screening. For example, should this information be included in an after-visit summary? What information, if any, should be shared with the patient's primary care provider?

Reporting and Evaluation

Once screening begins, it is critical to evaluate SDOH collection and intervention. In order to do so, the stakeholder groups need to develop and identify metrics/measures to monitor the collection and intervention processes. The team should set target goals and track progress in order to evaluate success.

Some key metrics include collection rates for SDOH overall, collection rates for each domain, screen positive rates for each domain, decline rates, and the number of referrals.

Other Considerations

Oftentimes it is challenging to launch a new screening enterprise-wide, and it is much more feasible to conduct pilot screening in a designated area, ideally one which might be particularly invested in this work with resources to address the issues identified. The data and lessons learned from the pilot can then be applied to enhance the screening process in that area and/or applied to the next area of implementation.

To support the processes created, a policy should be developed by the SDOH workgroup. This policy can be referenced to reinforce the work and should be reviewed and updated regularly as SDOH implementation is streamlined.

A Specialty Hospital Example

In a pilot study that took place at a rheumatology and orthopedic specialty hospital, a pediatric SDOH workgroup utilized a screening tool adapted from the WE CARE Screener [19], the PRAPARE Tool,[3] and a resource booklet; and an intervention process was developed. Nurses were trained to disseminate the screener and provide resources and/or social work referrals as appropriate.

The 10-item paper screener in English and Spanish with multiple choice and open-ended questions was disseminated over a 5-week period to patients in the outpatient pediatric rheumatology and orthopedic areas. The screener assessed the following domains: childcare, employment, housing, food insecurity, education, utilities, violence at home, and income-related needs. For each domain, the screener asked if the parent would like information. For housing and food insecurity, it asked if the need was an emergency, and if yes, a referral would be made to a social worker. If the patient screened in on violence at home, the family would be automatically referred to social work. Nurses introduced the screener to parents/guardians of patients using a standardized script. Families who identified a need were provided with the resource(s) and/or referred to a social worker. An analysis was conducted comparing patients with private insurance (PR) to those with public insurance (PU).

(continued)

[3] https://prapare.org/. Last visited: 04-21-2023

Of 451 surveys administered (98% English, 2% Spanish, patient age range 1–21 years), 276 surveys were completed (61%). Of this group, 50% were PU, and 50% PR. When asked about annual income, 32% declined, 7% were unsure, 33% indicated $100,000+, and 28% reported income of <$100,000.

Results showed the highest need reported need was employment, while utilities yielded the highest percentage requesting resources/referrals. When analyzed by insurance payers, PU respondents consistently reported higher needs across domains, with the largest differences being employment and education. The highest number of resources/referrals provided were for childcare and utilities.

The workgroup concluded that the implementation of this pilot increased the number of patients consistently screened for SDOH needs and subsequent provision of resources; however, there was still much work to be done to fully integrate screening into practice. For one, the screening only reached 22% of patients, which points to barriers to screening every patient, which in part may be due to the paper aspect of the screening. Of the group that completed the screening, 39% marked a decline to the entire survey. In addition, feedback from nursing staff pointed to concerns around stigma and families not answering questions truthfully, the time added on to rooming, and concerns around follow-up with the patient once a need has been identified.

The workgroup felt that adopting SDOH screening electronically and integrating it into the organization's EHR would help address many of the concerns from the pilot. This was adopted a year later, and the workgroup is in the process of evaluating electronic implementation.

References

1. Magnan S. Social determinants of health 101 for health care: five plus five. NAM perspectives. 2017.
2. Health SDo. Healthy People 2030, U.S. Department of Health and Human Services, Office of Disease Prevention and Health Promotion. https://health.gov/healthypeople/priority-areas/social-determinants-health. Accessed 21 Apr 2023.
3. 2023 HP. Social Determinants of Health Workgroup: Healthy People 2030, U.S. Department of Health and Human Services, Office of Disease Prevention and Health Promotion. https://health.gov/healthypeople/about/workgroups/social-determinants-health-workgroup. Accessed 21 Apr 2023.
4. Centers for Medicare & Medicaid Services DoHaHS. Inpatient Prospective Payment Systems. 2022. Contract No.: 2022–26986.
5. Services CfMaM. Table IX.E-01. The Hospital Commitment to Health Equity Measures Five Attestations. https://www.gnyha.org/wp-content/uploads/2022/08/CMS-FY23-IPPS-Table-IXE-01-FINAL.pdf. Accessed 21 Apr 2023.
6. R3 Report: The Joint Commission. 2022. https://www.jointcommission.org/-/media/tjc/documents/standards/r3-reports/r3_disparities_july2022-6-20-2022.pdf. Accessed 21 Apr 2023.
7. Olmsted MG, Powell R, Murphy J, Bell D, Stanley M, Sanchez RT et al. Methodology: U.S. News & World Report Best Children's Hospitals 2022–23. 2022. https://health.usnews.com/media/best-hospitals/BCH_Methodology_2022-23.pdf. Accessed 21 Apr 2023.
8. AHA Data. AHA Annual Survey Database™ The Most Credible and Consistent Data about the Nation's Hospitals [Internet]. AHA Data & Insights. https://www.ahadata.com/aha-annual-survey-database. Accessed 21 Apr 2023.
9. 2021 AHA Annual Survey American Hospital Association. AHA Data & Insights. 2021. https://www.ahadata.com/system/files/media/file/2022/11/2022-AHA-Annual-Survey-Questionnaire-Final.pdf. Accessed 21 Apr 2023.
10. Waas D. Screening for social needs: guiding care teams to engage patients. American Hospital Association; 2019.
11. Schoenthaler A, Hassan I, Fiscella K. The time is now: fostering relationship-centered discussions about patients' social determinants of health. Patient Educ Couns. 2019;102(4):810–4.
12. Medicare Cf, Services M. The accountable health communities health-related social needs screening tool: AHC Screening Tool. 2019. https://innovation.cms.gov/files/worksheets/ahcm-screeningtool.pdf. Accessed 21 Apr 2023.

13. Cartier YFF, Gottlieb L. Screening tools comparison tables2018. https://sirenetwork.ucsf.edu/tools-resources/resources/screening-tools-comparison-tables. Accessed 21 Apr 2023.
14. The Hunger Vital Sign: Children's Health Watch. https://childrenshealthwatch.org/public-policy/hunger-vital-sign/. Accessed 21 Apr 2023.
15. Hager ER, Quigg AM, Black MM, Coleman SM, Heeren T, Rose-Jacobs R, et al. Development and validity of a 2-item screen to identify families at risk for food insecurity. Pediatrics. 2010;126(1):e26–32.
16. Services CfMM. USING Z CODES: The Social Determinants of Health (SDOH) Data Journey to Better Outcomes: Centers for Medicare & Medicaid Services. https://www.cms.gov/files/document/zcodes-infographic.pdf. Accessed 21 Apr 2023.
17. ICD-10-CM Coding for Social Determinants of Health. 2022. https://www.aha.org/system/files/2018-04/value-initiative-icd-10-code-social-determinants-of-health.pdf. Accessed 21 Apr 2023.
18. Social Determinants of Health Information Exchange Toolkit: Office of the National Coordinator for Health Information Technology of the U.S. Department of Health and Human Services. https://www.healthit.gov/sites/default/files/2023-02/Social%20Determinants%20of%20Health%20Information%20Exchange%20Toolkit%202023_508.pdf. Accessed 21 Apr 2023.
19. The WE CARE Model: Boston Medical Center. https://www.bmc.org/pediatrics-primary-care/we-care/we-care-model. Accessed 21 Apr 2023.

13 The Impact of a Global Health Pandemic, Telehealth, and the Digital Divide

The Impact of COVID-19 on the Rheumatology Care Experience

The COVID-19 pandemic brought about numerous challenges for people with rheumatic conditions. Several studies looked at the experiences of patients with rheumatic diseases during the pandemic and found that patients experienced anxiety, sadness, isolation, and uncertainty coupled with fear of contracting COVID-19 [1–3]. Early in the pandemic, some patients had to stop or delay taking hydroxychloroquine due to medication shortages and no prescription renewal due to an increased demand for this medication as it was believed to be an effective treatment for COVID-19 [4]. The medication has since been proven to be ineffective [5, 6].

Patients also changed their behaviors related to their treatments during the pandemic. In one study that looked at treatment adherence, 20% of participants either spaced out or stopped their treatments, especially biological therapies. 63% of these patients stopped their medications due to fear of contracting COVID, and almost half of them changed their routine without telling their physician. Regardless of medication changes, 37% of patients reported worsening symptoms, i.e., pain and fatigue [3]. Many patients experienced interruptions in the delivery of healthcare, where their appointments were canceled or postponed. Patients

J. Rose-Smith et al., *The Psychosocial Impact of Rheumatic Conditions*, https://doi.org/10.1007/978-3-031-95338-5_13

were also concerned about communication with their healthcare team and reduced access to rheumatology care [7, 8].

A major shift in the care experience for patients was the switch to telemedicine appointments. In a study that surveyed rheumatologists worldwide between April and May 2020, the majority (82%) of these doctors changed to telehealth appointments, with 34% postponing all visits [9]. Another study reported a 65% decrease in outpatient visits, and of the in-person visits, strict social distancing guidelines such as masks and gloves were enforced. In 70% of cases, rheumatologists used telemedicine appointments, and in most cases, telemedicine was delivered through phone calls or emails which was not sustainable for long-term care [10].

A Rheumatology Specialty Hospital Study

According to the study "The Psychosocial Impact of the COVID-19 Pandemic on the Rheumatology Patient Experience," conducted in 2020, researchers sought to understand the psychosocial and emotional impact of the COVID-19 pandemic on people living with rheumatic illnesses. Furthermore, they aimed to learn about the types of psychosocial support and resources patients with rheumatic illnesses, and their loved ones need to better manage and cope with their rheumatic conditions during the pandemic [11].

Using a 95-item online survey in English and Spanish with a Likert scale and open-ended nationally disseminated questions, the survey assessed physical and mental health, illness management, access to care, social environment, and resources. The Patient Health Questionnaire-4 (PHQ-4) and the Hospital Anxiety and Depression Scale (HADS) were used to measure mental health status.

Patients in this sample were primarily diagnosed with lupus (SLE, NPSLE) and Arthritis (RA, PsA, OA, AS, JRA, SpA) with a mean of 13 years since diagnosis. Over half (63%) reported a flare since the pandemic, and 16% reported having COVID-19. Only 19% reported no changes to their care during the pandemic, and one-third (33%) indicated that their care switched to telehealth visits or had their appointments postponed (19%).

76% reported a change in their mood and/or emotional health (ECs), with 81% attributing this change to the pandemic. More than half of the respondents (54%) scored "borderline or abnormal" on the HADS Anxiety score, and 43% scored the same on the HADS Depression score. Lastly, most participants (82%) responded that they sometimes (37%), usually (26%), or always (19%) "feel isolated from others."

A comparative analysis was conducted for those who reported a change in emotional health (ECs) vs. those who did not (NECs). Significant differences were found with a higher proportion of patients reporting a negative emotion change indicating they switched to telehealth, received mental health services, took medication for their mental health needs, and started counseling. Similarly, they reported more contact with their rheumatologist or other health professionals, higher PHQ-4 and HADS scores, and more difficulty maintaining social relationships. Almost half of these patients indicated a desire for support programs to cope with their condition.

When asked about the types of resources that would be most helpful to this sample overall, virtual programs on coping and managing an illness, virtual programs on managing emotional health, and mental health resources were the highest reported.

The researchers also conducted a thematic analysis of open-ended questions for patients. When asked about what they would change about their care experiences, themes included better communication with the healthcare team, improved access to care, and information about risks due to their rheumatic condition. When asked about what social workers and other providers could do differently to best meet their needs, themes pointed to increasing outreach and check-ins, facilitating connection with others, and more information and education. Patients were also asked about the impact of the pandemic on them and their loved ones, and most respondents underscored social isolation, fear, mental health, stress, and adjusting to the new normal. One person shared, "I live alone. Completely alone. I can go days without hearing a human voice. My antidepressant dosage was doubled twice during these months but not much difference."

The findings of this particular study indicate that the healthcare team should be especially cognizant of anxiety, depression, and isolation concerns in patients with rheumatic conditions in this era of the COVID-19 pandemic. It points to the need for the care team to find more ways to be more accessible to their patients in a post-pandemic world. There is a need for more ways to stay connected to patients beyond the traditional in-person visit. Lastly, it underscores the need to assess and address mental health issues that patients with rheumatic conditions are already particularly prone to.

Telehealth and the Digital Divide in Rheumatology

According to the Federal Communications Commission (FCC), "approximately 19 million Americans—6 percent of the population—still lack access to fixed broadband service at threshold speeds. In rural areas, nearly one-fourth of the population—14.5 million people—lack access to this service" [12]. Increasing evidence shows that digital access and Internet connectivity have an impact on health outcomes, with public health advocates identifying this as a social determinant of health. According to Saeed and Masters, low digital/health literacy, poor access to the Internet, lack of support resources, and skepticism of new technological advancements contribute to this "digital divide," in which "technology and internet utilization patterns differ by race/ethnicity and socioeconomic lines" [13]. Proposed solutions include "advocating for improved internet access, providing IT support, advertising technologies to patients, and educating patients on the benefits of these technologies" [13].

The onset of the COVID-19 pandemic brought special attention to the digital divide as daily life, such as work and school, moved to online platforms. The pandemic opened the doors for accessing and advancing telehealth as individuals were encouraged to stay at home to prevent the spread of illness. This was even more important for patients with rheumatic conditions who are in immunocompromised states. Studies have looked at telehealth in rheumatology care since the pandemic, and many have underscored positive findings related to health outcomes and the patient and clinician experience. According to Matsumoto and Barton, who specifically looked at telerheumatology studies for RA, telehealth visits were "non-inferior to in-person visits and are often more time and cost-effective for patients" [14]. They found in the literature that patients generally found telehealth to be beneficial and convenient, but this was also largely dependent on the patient's preference, noting that there is no "one-size-fits-all" approach. The authors also found that the largest barrier was not being able to conduct a physical exam [14]. Other studies support the use of virtual visits for stable disease conditions and follow-up appointments [15].

In a study that looked at rheumatology patient and provider perceptions of telehealth, researchers found most patients found telehealth appointments more convenient but not necessarily equally or more effective. There was a strong preference for face-to-face consultations for both providers and patients, and the researchers found that telemedicine was inappropriate for initial diagnosis. This study found no differences in telemedicine preferences between rheumatic disease groups; however, patients with inflammatory arthritis were significantly more confident in receiving a quick response from their rheumatology care team and higher ratings for feeling medically secure compared to other, more rare rheumatic diseases, such as lupus and Sjogren's. This raised concerns about telehealth possibly contributing to the existing inequities in the treatment of rarer rheumatic conditions [15].

Researchers Jackson and Danila discuss healthcare disparities in telemedicine for people with rheumatic conditions. With its widespread adoption during the pandemic, access to rheumatology had the potential to expand; however, disparities persisted in vulnerable groups, including racial and ethnic minorities, those with lower socioeconomic status, and older adults who have underutilized these services [15]. Barriers to telemedicine in these populations include a lack of high-speed Internet, costly communication devices, rural locations, and level of digital literacy [14, 15]. A study by George, Danila, and colleagues found that rheumatology patients who were older, of Black or Hispanic descent, and of lower socioeconomic status living in rural areas were most likely to cancel visits. Despite telehealth growing to more than

40% of follow-up visits in the study, those who were older adults of low socioeconomic status and residing in rural areas were less likely to use telehealth [15].

In a pilot study at a rheumatology and orthopedic specialty clinic, which surveyed a total of 164 patients on their use of telehealth services, 43% of patients reported having one to two visits (25%) and three or more visits (18%). When asked about the reasons telehealth would be difficult for them, the top responses included the following: health needs would be difficult to address over telehealth (18%), difficulty using technology (logging in, starting the call, turning on the camera, etc.) (16%), access to a large enough device (computer, smartphone, or laptop) with a camera (14%), unclear how to make a telehealth appointment (14%), some other reason (13%), and concerns about privacy or security (10%). Other reasons included a preference for in-person interaction, the need for a physician exam or labs, and being unfamiliar with technology. When asked about how willing they would be to use telehealth in the future, 60% of patients reported that they were moderately willing (27%), very willing (14%), and extremely willing (19%). Lastly, the researchers looked at open-ended feedback from patients related to telehealth. Themes that were categorized as telehealth advantages included an overall willingness to use telehealth, reduced travel time, convenience, and less of a need to walk. Themes categorized as barriers included lack of familiarity with technology and poor Internet connection.

These findings reinforce the need for rheumatology care providers to be especially cognizant of disparities related to telehealth usage and access, ensuring that its use does not exacerbate existing disparities. It also points to a need to provide interventions to address these barriers.

Strategies to Address Telehealth Disparities

Possible solutions to address disparities in telehealth include interventions with patients to enhance digital literacy, including access to telehealth technology, support, and patient education on how to use technology [15]. This may require coaching from members of the healthcare team, whether they are patient services liasons, registration staff, social workers, or nurses. Materials such as informational tip sheets with step-by-step instructions can be particularly useful to patients and should be at an appropriate reading level. For more information on health literacy, please see Chaps. 7 and 10. It's also critical to have this information and in-person support available to patients in their preferred language.

Contents of a sample tipsheet for patients on preparing for their telehealth appointment during the COVID-19 pandemic are shared below:

Telehealth/Telemedicine Tip Sheet

Benefits of Telehealth/Telemedicine

- Limiting physical contact reduces everyone's exposure to COVID-19.
- Telehealth visits can address health issues wherever patients are, even from the comfort of home.
- Cuts down on commuting, travel in bad weather, time off from work, and need for childcare.
- Using virtual healthcare tools can shorten wait times to see a provider and expand the range of access to specialists who live further away.
- Ability for providers to do the following in a safe and accessible way:
  - Coach and support for patients managing chronic health conditions.
  - Review labs, X-rays, and other relevant results for new patients and existing patients.
  - Review medications and treatment plans and provide follow-up care.

Preparing for Appointments

Telemedicine can be defined as the use of technology (computers, video, phone, messaging) by a medical professional to diagnose and treat patients in a remote location.

Preparing for Telemedicine Appointments

- Pick your medium—call your doctor's office to ensure you can get into your patient portals.
    - Ensure your Internet connection is reliable.
  - Have the phone as a backup, and test the sound.
    - Ask how long the appointment will be and how you should prepare.
- If you are using a non-health app like Zoom or FaceTime, test it out beforehand with family or friends so they can tell you how it looks.
- Invite a family member or friend to be a part of the appointment to assist with technology or to have an extra pair of eyes and ears to help you take in the information to minimize distractions.
- Consider if you need a language interpreter or other assistance, such as closed captioning or other resources to support your communication needs.
- Set the stage:
  - Find a quiet space with minimal interruptions.
  - Turn off your TV and noisy devices.
  - Sit in front of a solid-colored wall if possible.
  - Try to use a well-lit area. Position lighting close to you.
  - Have a torch light on hand to illuminate areas the doctor may want to see.
  - Have a thermometer, scale, tissue, cotton swab, pen, and paper nearby.
  - Have a path available to walk or stand up in case the doctor wants you to demonstrate or assess movement.

- Write down your questions and track your symptoms in a journal or app.
- Have your medications handy.
- Discuss follow-up:
  - Repeat instructions or recommendations from the doctor, i.e., "You said to change my dose of prednisone to X twice a day for the next week." This will help clear up any misunderstanding.
  - Ask important follow-up questions: "Will you be sending me the new treatment plan via email?" "Will you be sending out my new prescription to the pharmacy?" etc.
- Remember: Don't delay care in-person!

Preparing for In-person Appointments

- Call to ask what safety precautions your provider is taking to avoid the spread of COVID-19. Healthcare systems and doctors' offices are putting safety measures in place to keep you safe if you need an in-person office visit:
  - Reduced number of in-person visits.
  - Scheduled additional time between appointments to minimize contact between patients and for cleaning exam rooms.
  - Adjusted setup of waiting room to accommodate social distancing—some doctors allow people to wait in their cars until they are ready to see them.
  - Use of face masks.
  - Limitations on the number of people with a patient and inpatient visitor:
    - Negotiating elevator.
    - Waiting rooms.
    - Physical exam.
    - X-rays.
    - Infusions.
    - Blood draws.

Conclusion

Many valuable and lasting lessons were learned from the impact of COVID-19 on the rheumatology care experience with advances in telehealth, attention to disparities in the digital divide, and the development of strategies for addressing emergent needs.

According to Jackson and Danila, other strategies for addressing disparities include integrating electronic patient-reported outcomes (PRO) for telemedicine visits, where telehealth technologies could enable PRO collection between visits or during telemedicine visits. Studies in which these applications have been utilized have reported success with older adult patients. Furthermore, adopting eConsult services, where a provider can share health information with a specialist who can provide clinical advice without seeing the patient, can help address rheumatology shortages in rural areas [15].

Addressing these challenges by utilizing some of these strategies can help bridge the gap to promote more equitable access to rheumatology care.

References

1. Michaud K, Wipfler K, Shaw Y, Simon TA, Cornish A, England BR, et al. Experiences of patients with rheumatic diseases in the United States during early days of the COVID-19 pandemic. ACR Open Rheumatol. 2020;2(6):335–43.
2. van Zanten J, Fenton SAM, Brady S, Metsios GS, Duda JL, Kitas GD. Mental health and psychological wellbeing in rheumatoid arthritis during COVID-19 - can physical activity help? Mediterr J Rheumatol. 2020;31(Suppl 2):284–7.
3. López-Medina C, Ladehesa-Pineda L, Gómez-García I, Puche-Larrubia M, Sequí-Sabater JM, Armenteros-Ortiz P, et al. Treatment adherence during the COVID-19 pandemic and the impact of confinement on disease activity and emotional status: a survey in 644 rheumatic patients. Joint Bone Spine. 2021;88(2):105085.
4. Abu-Zaid MH, Aly HM, Moshrif A, Abdeldaim DE, El-Ghobashy N. Hydroxychloroquine non-availability during COVID-19 pandemic and its relation to anxiety level and disease activity in rheumatoid arthritis and lupus patients: a cross-sectional study. Egypt Rheumatol Rehabil. 2022;49(1):17.

5. Hennekens CH, Rane M, Solano J, Alter S, Johnson H, Krishnaswamy S, et al. Updates on Hydroxychloroquine in prevention and treatment of COVID-19. Am J Med. 2022;135(1):7–9.
6. Coronavirus disease (COVID-19): hydroxychloroquine: World Health Organization. 2020. https://www.who.int/news-room/questions-and-answers/item/coronavirus-disease-(covid-19)-hydroxychloroquine. Accessed 28 2023.
7. Sloan M, Gordon C, Harwood R, Lever E, Wincup C, Bosley M, et al. The impact of the COVID-19 pandemic on the medical care and health-care behaviour of patients with lupus and other systemic autoimmune diseases: a mixed methods longitudinal study. Rheumatol Adv Pract. 2021;5(1):rkaa072.
8. Opinc A, Brzezińska O, Makowska J. The impact of COVID-19 and healthcare system changes on the well-being of rheumatic patients. Reumatologia. 2021;59(2):73–84.
9. Mehta B, Jannat-Khah D, Fontana MA, Moezinia CJ, Mancuso CA, Bass AR, et al. Impact of COVID-19 on vulnerable patients with rheumatic disease: results of a worldwide survey. RMD Open. 2020;6(3):e001378.
10. Ziadé N, Hmamouchi I, El Kibbi L, Abdulateef N, Halabi H, Abutiban F, et al. The impact of COVID-19 pandemic on rheumatology practice: a cross-sectional multinational study. Clin Rheumatol. 2020;39(11):3205–13.
11. Flores M, Toral P, Horton R, Batterman A, Seehaus M, Kleinman J, Rose J. The psychosocial impact of the COVID-19 pandemic on the rheumatology patient experience: abstract number: 0266. Arthritis Rheumatol. 2021;73:541–2.
12. Eighth Broadband Progress Report: Federal Communications Commission. https://www.fcc.gov/reports-research/reports/broadband-progress-reports/eighth-broadband-progress-report#:~:text=Notwithstanding%20this%20progress%2C%20the%20Report,lack%20access%20to%20this%20service. Accessed 28 2023.
13. Saeed SA, Masters RM. Disparities in health care and the digital divide. Curr Psychiatry Rep. 2021;23(9):61.
14. Matsumoto RA, Barton JL. Telerheumatology: before, during, and after a global pandemic. Curr Opin Rheumatol. 2021;33(3):262–9.
15. Jackson LE, Danila MI. Healthcare disparities in telemedicine for rheumatology care. Curr Opin Rheumatol. 2022;34(3):171–8.

Engaging Patients in Research: Incorporating the Patient Perspective

14

Strategies to Optimize Patient Recruitment: Building Trust and Engagement

Patient participation in clinical trials and research studies is invaluable to the field of rheumatology to help advance knowledge and treatments and improve health outcomes; however, it is well-known that recruiting and retaining participants is a challenge. To optimize patient engagement in research, there are several core skills which can be used, including the use of empathy and attunement, as well as fostering feelings of trust, safety, and respect. Furthermore, communication tools are often used in social work practice that can be leveraged to build trust and rapport with patients, opening the door to engagement in research.

Exploring Empathy, Attunement, Trust, Safety, and Respect

Empathy "Empathy is one of the fundamental tools of the therapeutic relationship between the carers and their patients and it has been proven that its contribution is vital to better health outcomes." [1]. Think back to a time when someone appeared to understand your situation or point of view and how that made you feel. That is empathy—it's the capacity to be aware of another's

J. Rose-Smith et al., *The Psychosocial Impact of Rheumatic Conditions*, https://doi.org/10.1007/978-3-031-95338-5_14

experience and understand it. It is not just about labeling an emotion, but it's also about putting yourself in that person's shoes and imagining the feelings that person may be having.

Attunement Attunement takes it one step further. It's the state of recognizing, understanding, and engaging with someone's emotional state. It allows us to build relationships because it involves tuning into someone's emotional state and offering genuine efforts to understand their emotions. For example, if a patient is distressed, they are less likely to listen to what you are saying when you approach them. Healthcare providers and researchers may often work from a script or assessment guide when approaching patients. As a result, if a patient feels you are not genuinely interested in them, then they will be less engaged and less inclined to listen. Showing you care about and support a person's situation will help with relationship-building.

Creating Safety, Trust, and Respect People living with rheumatic conditions are coping with a variety of physical and emotional challenges such as isolation and feeling misunderstood. Empathy and attunement are crucial skills for creating safety, trust, and respect in a patient encounter. People are more likely to be open and willing to share their thoughts and listen to you when they feel safe and respected. Experiencing another person as empathic and caring facilitates communication and trust. To help you connect with the patient, pay special attention to the patient's needs at the moment. You can increase the likelihood of a patient participating in your study by recognizing their unique needs [2].

Engaging Patients for Readiness The definition of engagement is the process of establishing a genuine rapport while creating a pleasant emotional connection. How do we engage patients to promote readiness to participate in our study? When approaching patients about research participation, it is important to establish rapport while creating an emotional connection. Engaging a patient in a working relationship is the first step to helping a person feel comfortable for and ready to participate in your research study. There are some key ingredients needed to be successful at engagement. We want you to think about this as a recipe, as all these core skills together make the recipe complete. Below are some specific tools and techniques for you to consider, as key ingredients for successful engagement. These skills are all foundational to social work practice [3, 4].

Ingredients for Engagement

- **Respect, Dignity, and Cultural Sensitivity**. It's important to ask how the patient would like to be referred to. Use appropriate gender pronouns as identified by the patient.
- **Confidentiality:** Ensure confidentiality by being discreet and giving privacy to the patient, even as it relates to finding a confidential area to speak openly, when possible.
- **Commitment:** Show an interest in the patient and the study. If the patient feels you care about the work, they will be more likely to participate.
- **Active listening:** Involves going beyond hearing what a person is saying but trying to understand the meaning and intent behind what they are sharing. It requires one to be an active participant in the communication exchange.

When interviewing patients, it's important to ask questions slowly so you can really absorb what the patient is communicating. This may often be a challenge when meeting patients in time pressured situations or if the patient is hesitant about participating in research. If you are feeling nervous, you may be thinking about the next question to ask and may miss critical information being shared by the patient. Below are additional engagement tips to support your communication.

Engagement: Quick Tips

- **Be professional and warm**—approach or call the patient with a warm, friendly, professional greeting.
- **Don't rush**—allow the patient to take in what you are saying and respond to you. It's important to be familiar with the information and share what you can in your own words.
- **Give specific information** about who you are and why you are approaching or calling the patient. That's important because that already starts adding some of that personal touch to the patient encounter.
- **Invite the patient to participate** and offer to follow up by phone if they need more time to consider the information presented.
- **Be sensitive** to the patients' immediate concerns, for example, patients may be in pain, upset, and/or tired.
- **Be aware and tune in** to how the patient is responding to you. What cues are they providing? Are they quiet, ignoring you, or are they interested?
- **Be mindful of nonverbal cues**—yours and the patient. Your tone of voice and body language are important and set the tone for how you approach the patient and how they respond to you.

Engagement Script

Below is a brief script you may want to modify that puts some of the engagement quick tips in practice:

- *Hello, my name is_____. Are you [Patient's Name]?*
- *"How are you today?"* (Pause, and let the patient answer)
- *"May I speak with you for a moment?" (Pause.) "I am a research coordinator here at the hospital, and I'm working with Dr. ___ on a research study."* (Explain the project in a few short sentences.)
- *"I'm not sure if you would be interested, but may I share some information about the study with you?"*

Remembering to pause is key because it helps the patient, and you gather your thoughts throughout the exchange. The last bullet is critical; this is the invitation to participate—it offers the patient a choice whether to engage in the study and or share potential concerns about their participation.

Active listening is a fundamental component of the interpersonal communication skills shared above. It is a way of listening and responding to another person that improves mutual understanding. It helps the receiver to feel more at ease and communicate more easily, openly, and honestly. Below are some additional guidelines to support your engagement of participants in research studies using active listening.

Active Listening Tips

- **Practice Mindful listening:** A type of active listening is mindful listening. It's a way of hearing what a person is saying to you without judgment, criticism, or interruption. Some ways to demonstrate this are by your use of eye contact, using open body language, and using a welcoming vocal style.
- **Use Minimal Encouragers:** These are small signals that let the speaker know you are listening and understanding. Words like "uh-huh," "yes," "go on," "tell me more," or "I'm listening" encourage the speaker to continue sharing with minimum interruption and show that you are listening or engaged.
- **Use Teach-Back:** Have the person repeat back or paraphrase what was said to them, in order to assess their understanding of the research study. For example, you might say, "I want to ensure you understood all of the information I shared today, can you tell me in your own words what you heard." For more information on how to use the teach-back method, refer to Chap. 4 [5].
- **Ask open-ended questions:** Open-ended questions are questions that invite a person to share more and cannot be answered with a simple "yes" or "no." They often require a person to elaborate more on what they are being asked.
  - Open-ended questions start with: "how," "what," or "tell me."

- **Close-ended questions:** Close-ended questions are different than open-ended questions because they don't typically elicit more than a "yes or no" response. They are helpful in gathering focused information needed, like dates, numbers, or one-word answers.
  - Close ended questions start with: "have," "did," or "are."

Here are some examples of **Open-Ended vs. Closed Ended Questions** you may consider using when communicating about your research study.

Open-ended questions	Closed-ended questions
What brings you here today?	**Have** you ever heard of this research study?
Tell me about your illness and treatment plan?	**Are** you interested in hearing more?
What do you know about research studies?	**Did** you understand what the research coordinator shared?

Engaging Diverse Multicultural Populations in Research: Why?

The US population is getting increasingly more diverse each year. Based on the 2020 Census, beyond 2030, the US population is projected to grow slowly, age considerably, and become more racially and ethnically diverse. In 2023, there are 334 million people in the USA, and in 2058, The US Census Bureau projects we will cross 400 million [6]. In 2045 immigration is projected to be the primary driver of population growth for the country, and there will be an increase in diversity across all racial groups. In 2012 the Hispanic/Latinx population became the largest minority, and within the last 20 years, the Asian and Pacific Islander population nearly doubled to 23 million [7]. It's projected that by 2045 people of color will become the majority.

As we discuss engaging diverse populations in research, it's important to acknowledge the concept of implicit bias, which affects all of us. This refers to attitudes or stereotypes that impact our actions and decision-making in an unconscious manner. These biases operate outside of one's own awareness and may impact our feelings, thoughts, and attitudes about others based on characteristics such as gender, language, race, and age. These associations develop over the course of a lifetime starting at a young age. Please refer to Chap. 5 to learn more about this concept.

In research, we may very consciously be seeking patients who fit specific study criteria which may unintentionally alienate others. Some examples of exclusion criteria may be people who are pregnant or people who have certain comorbidities. In-person recruitment may also be impacted by bias when the recruiter assumes a prospective participant would comply with the research protocols based on the recruiter's lived experience with specific populations.

Case Scenario *Tim is a new research coordinator for Dr. Blume, the Principal Investigator on a clinical trial for a rheumatoid arthritis study that is actively recruiting participants. Tim overhears patient R.O. speaking to his wife with a Spanish accent. Tim became concerned that the patient would have a difficult time understanding the research protocols and assumed it would be too difficult to engage him, so he hesitated to reach out to the patient after his medical appointment. Tim learns later that R.O. is a very active patient advocate in the RA community and has participated in past studies. This led to a missed opportunity to engage the patient due to Tim's own assumptions and biases.*

Call to Action: Diversifying Research

The inclusion of communities of color and diverse populations in research is consistent with the national climate of our country and accrediting bodies who are seeking intentional inclusion of diverse and multicultural populations to assess and address healthcare disparities. For example, the National Institutes of Health released the NIH Minority Health and Health Disparities Strategic Plan 2021–2025 that reinforces that NIH is committed to inclusivity in clinical trial research [8, 9].

According to the NIH, historically, clinical trials did not always recruit participants reflective of people most affected by the disease. This created gaps in our understanding of diseases and conditions, preventive factors, and treatment effectiveness across populations, which ultimately impede the quality of healthcare decision-making, optimal treatment responses, and development of more effective interventions. The NIH recommends that clinicians and researchers should carefully examine inclusion and exclusion criteria to ensure that the trial doesn't unintentionally exclude groups that may benefit the most from findings [10].

In the USA, individuals participating in rheumatology research are more likely to be non-Hispanic White despite patients from minority communities having a higher prevalence of rheumatic conditions such as SLE and being more likely to develop more severe manifestations. For example, in a study that looked at race/ethnicity of patients participating in randomized control trials (RCTs), White patients comprised 33% of prevalent SLE cases at the time and 51% of those enrolled in RCTs while Black/African American patients comprised 43% of prevalent SLE cases but only represented 14% of RCT enrollees [11].

Impact of Culture

There are several aspects that can affect patient engagement in research, and one of these factors is culture. We introduced the concept of culture in Chap. 5. When we think about culture, we need to think about how it intersects with so many other aspects of our patients' lives.

We want to approach patients with respect, dignity, and cultural sensitivity, and one way we can do that is by practicing from a stance of professional curiosity—not making assumptions about how a person identifies. To be inclusive of LGBTQIA+ patients (and all patients), for example, it's important to ask open-ended questions such as: "How would you like me to address you?" Someone may have a chosen name that is different from their legal name, or their pronouns may be different than what you expect. The best way to make sure you're not assuming is to ask.

Instead of guessing who is accompanying a patient to their appointment (a parent, a brother), ask "who did you bring with you today?" For more communication strategies for promoting an LGBTQIA+ inclusive environment, see Chap. 7.

As mentioned in Chap. 5, culture can be described as the "lens" through which you view the world, which impacts how one thinks, feels, expresses themselves, and behaves. It defines what is "normal" for a person and influences a person's health beliefs and their approach to healthcare and treatment. For some patients it's important to consult family members about any new treatments being considered—whether a partner, a parent, or a family "matriarch" or "patriarch"—prior to following through. Culture can also influence a person's view of their disease. For example, not all lupus patients think illness is caused by a disruption in their immune system–a Western scientific view—but they may think that it is spiritual in nature—a personalistic view. Thus, we want to be sensitive towards others' thought processes about what is causing their illness and how that influences how patients cope with and manage their illness. These types of factors can therefore affect one's hesitance or inclination to participate in research.

To address culture when engaging patients in research, it's critical to practice from a stance of cultural humility, as referenced in Chap. 5. By seeing patients as experts on their own lives and approaching our work with a commitment to actively engage in a partnership with diverse individuals and groups, we create a bridge to understanding and mutual respect. Given that historical mistrust of healthcare and research is common in communities of color—as seen with the COVID-19 pandemic and vaccine hesitancy [12]—we want to foster relationships with patients in which they are partners instead of test subjects.

Stereotyping Versus Generalizing: Applying to Patient Recruitment to Combat Bias

Thinking about culture and implicit bias, it's valuable to discuss the difference between stereotyping and generalizing and how this can be applied during the patient recruitment process:

- Stereotyping: Assumption without further exploration = HARMFUL.
- Generalizing: Initial assumption followed up by curious exploration.

It's important to challenge any biases or stereotypes we may hold, as they can create barriers to meaningful engagement. We should avoid making broad assumptions about people from specific cultural groups. Instead, we should focus on observing, questioning our assumptions, and then exploring further.

Below are some examples of how we can challenge our initial biases:

Stereotyping: assumption without further exploration = HARMFUL	Generalizing: initial assumption followed up by curious exploration
They are too old to do the required activities.	*They seem older than patients I have been enrolling. Let me check in with them about the study to hear what they think about participating.*
He can't understand—I hear him only speaking Spanish.	*I often hear him speaking Spanish. I wonder if he reads and understands English, however. If so, he would be able to fill out our survey. Let me ask.*
They are not the right fit for a focus group. They are Chinese and won't speak up.	*In my experience Chinese patients don't say much in focus groups. But I know that being "quiet" or "passive" is a stereotype in the Asian community. I will share this opportunity with them anyway and let them decide.*
As a single mother, she doesn't have time.	*I know she is a single mother of 3 children, but I should explore if she has an interest. She could have other support at home or child care arrangements I'm not aware of.*
They ambulate with a walker. It will be too difficult for them to stay longer than they need to.	*Although they ambulate with a device, perhaps they would find value in participating in the study and want to stay the extra time.*
Those people are not good at following up.	*What do I mean by "those people?" am I stereotyping a whole group of people based on perceived socioeconomic status? Race? Ethnicity? I need to change my mindset here.*

What should we do if we make a mistake with a patient? For example, if you make an incorrect assumption about how a patient identifies, it's crucial to acknowledge the mistake and offer a sincere apology immediately. Some possible phrases include: "I'm so sorry I assumed ____." Or, "that was my mistake" or "I didn't have all the information and I want to apologize for getting it wrong." It's important to address the error openly, rather than ignoring it and risk losing that relationship completely.

Barriers to Patient Participation

As we aim to engage diverse patients in research, it's important to acknowledge and be mindful of some of the very real barriers to participation. Sandhu and colleagues set out to identify barriers reported by patients that impact their ability to participate in clinical research and found that the top-ranked barriers were fear of associated risks, work responsibilities, and fear of discovering a serious illness [13]. Below are additional barriers to participation with proposed strategies to address these concerns:

- **Lack of awareness of clinical trials**: Patients are unaware of clinical trials, or do not know they may be eligible to participate. While we may believe our recruitment efforts are effective, we may not be reaching all eligible patients. Often, patients are either not referred to clinical trials appropriately or may not be referred at all by their treating clinicians, sometimes unintentionally.
  - **Ways to address this**: Bridge the gap between patient and researchers by hosting tailored informational/educational sessions on participation in research—covering why research is important, health disparities for specific disease groups, how to get involved, and including opportunities for questions. This can help demystify research for patients who may be hesitant because they did not know enough about the process and want to be able to make an informed decision.

- **Cost concerns**: Costs involved in participating in research can deter patients—such as not being able to afford transportation for what seems like an additional appointment, child care concerns, or even costs associated with meals if they have to be out of their homes for several hours.
  - **Ways to address this**: Work with your social work team to explore resources available, build in vouchers for transportation/meals, or add other incentives as appropriate in your study process, in order to address some of the costs associated with participating.
- **Language barriers**: The lack of bilingual staff and lack of study materials available in multiple languages can be a barrier to patient participation. Information may therefore be difficult to understand and consent cannot be obtained appropriately.
  - **Ways to address this**: Work with your language services team to ensure that educational materials about research are translated in the most common languages and either work in collaboration with a staff interpreter or hire bilingual research assistants certified for medical interpretation.
- **Health literacy concerns**: Some patients may have difficulty with reading, so it's important to pay attention to health literacy cues. Oftentimes study materials are complex and filled with unfamiliar medical jargon.
  - **Ways to address this**: Health literacy screening can assist with identifying one's needs. Create materials utilizing health literacy tools written at the sixth to eighth grade reading level as recommended by the AMA and NIH [14].
- **Historical mistrust**: Lack of trust in general due to a history of human rights violations especially in minority communities.
  - **Ways to address this:** Hire diverse research staff reflective of the community one is seeking to engage. Utilize communication strategies, build rapport with patients over time and explore concerns around patient participation in research. Communicate safeguards in place, emphasize patient autonomy, and ensure transparency of information.
- **Risk involved**: Patients who are clinically stable may feel that participation in a study is too risky since there is no guarantee that the treatment will make them feel better or improve their

health outcomes. Participation may negatively impact their quality of life.

   – **Ways to address this**: Engage in open conversation with patients around the risks and benefits to equip patients with the information they need to weigh the pros and cons and make a decision. Remember, ultimately this is the patient's decision and a patient should not feel forced to participate in research if they do not have the desire to do so.

If we don't address these barriers, this can lead to unintended marginalization or discrimination. A patient may not feel heard and instead feel isolated and disengaged. By incorporating strategies such as asking open-ended questions, ensuring equitable access to information, and connecting patients with resources like social work to address social concerns, we can better support their ability to participate in research. These approaches help create a more inclusive environment and remove potential barriers to participation.

Summary To summarize, as we aim to engage diverse populations in research, we should be aware of our own values, beliefs, and cultural norms. Remember it's best not to make assumptions. And when you are unsure, it's okay to ask. It's critical to address the barriers faced by patients: explore concerns in open discussions, and revisit your recruitment and educational materials to ensure they are patient-friendly and translated in multiple languages. Finally, understanding cultural diversity and applying these insights to engage patients in research is an ongoing journey. We're not expected to have all the answers, but it's essential to actively seek opportunities for learning and to practice cultural humility. Through mutual respect and understanding, we can create a partnership that empowers patients, fosters trust, and ensures that research is truly inclusive with representation from diverse communities.

References

1. Moudatsou M, Stavropoulou A, Philalithis A, Koukouli S. The role of empathy in health and social care professionals. Healthcare. 2020;8(1):26.
2. Wilkins CH, Edwards TL, Stroud M, Kennedy N, Jerome RN, Lawrence CE, et al. The recruitment innovation center: developing novel, person-centered strategies for clinical trial recruitment and retention. J Clin Transl Sci. 2021;5(1):e194.

3. Krist AH, Tong ST, Aycock RA, Longo DR. Engaging patients in decision-making and behavior change to promote prevention. Stud Health Technol Inform. 2017;240:284–302.
4. Duffett L. Patient engagement: what partnering with patient in research is all about. Thromb Res. 2017;150:113–20.
5. Talevski J, Wong Shee A, Rasmussen B, Kemp G, Beauchamp A. Teach-back: a systematic review of implementation and impacts. PLoS One. 2020;15(4):e0231350.
6. Vespa JE, Armstrong DM, Medina L. Demographic turning points for the United States: Population projections for 2020 to 2060. US Department of Commerce, Economics and Statistics Administration, US ...; 2018.
7. Budiman A, Ruiz NG. Key facts about Asian Americans, a diverse and growing population [Internet]. Pew Research Center. 2021. Available from: https://www.pewresearch.org/short-reads/2021/04/29/key-facts-about-asian-americans/
8. NIMHD. Strategic Plan. 2024. Available from: https://nimhd.nih.gov/about/strategic-plan/index.html
9. National Institutes of Health. Minority health and health disparities strategic plan 2021–2025. Bethesda Md Natl Inst Health. 2021.
10. NIMHD. Diversity and Inclusion in Clinical Trials. 2024. Available from: https://nimhd.nih.gov/resources/understanding-health-disparities/diversity-and-inclusion-in-clinical-trials.html
11. Falasinnu T, Chaichian Y, Bass MB, Simard JF. The representation of gender and race/ethnic groups in randomized clinical trials of individuals with systemic lupus erythematosus. Curr Rheumatol Rep. 2018;20(4):20. https://doi.org/10.1007/s11926-018-0728-2.
12. Quinn SC, Andrasik MP. Addressing vaccine hesitancy in BIPOC communities – toward trustworthiness, partnership, and reciprocity. N Engl J Med. 2021;385(2):97–100.
13. Sandhu VK, Duro T, Kamboj A, Salto L, Chiruvolu N. Barriers to enrollment in rheumatology research: who, what, where, when, and why? Cureus. 2022;14(7):e27235.
14. Rooney MK, Santiago G, Perni S, Horowitz DP, McCall AR, Einstein AJ, et al. Readability of patient education materials from high-impact medical journals: a 20-year analysis. J Patient Exp. 2021;8:2374373521998847.

Index

A
Accountable Health Communities Health-Related Social Needs Screening Tool, 128
Active listening, 153, 155, 156
Adherence, 61, 62
  condition-related factors and therapy-related factors, 65, 66
  healthcare system factors, 63
  patient-related factors, 64, 65
  physician factors, 64
  socioeconomic factors, 62, 63
  strategies to, 66–69
Adolescence, 91–93
Affordable Care Act, 25, 48
Agency for Healthcare Research and Quality (AHRQ), 27, 32
American College of Rheumatology (ACR), 73
Anxiety, rheumatic condition, 10–12
Attunement, 152

B
Beck depression inventory, 17
Bundle payments, 78

C
Care coordination, 75, 78
Care Everywhere, 74
Centers for Medicare and Medicaid Services (CMS), 122
Certified Electronic Health Record Technology (CEHRT), 57
Charla de Lupus (Lupus Chat)® Program, 92–94
Chronic illness, 61, 77, 87, 92
  and family experience, 89–92
Civil Rights Act, 49
Closed-ended questions, 156
Collaborative communication, 79
Collaborative culture, 80
Columbia Severity Scale (C-SSRS), 17
Combat bias, patient recruitment, 159–161
Commitment, 153
Communication, 77
Community resources, 81
Compliance, 61
  condition-related factors and therapy-related factors, 65, 66
  healthcare system factors, 63
  patient-related factors, 64, 65
  physician factors, 64
  socioeconomic factors, 62, 63

J. Rose-Smith et al., *The Psychosocial Impact of Rheumatic Conditions*, https://doi.org/10.1007/978-3-031-95338-5

Condition-related factors, 65, 66
Confidentiality, 153
Coping, 87, 92
Counter-stereotypic imaging, 117
COVID-19, rheumatology care, 139, 140
  rheumatology specialty hospital study, 140–142
Cultural competency, 38
Cultural factors, 38, 43
Cultural humility, 41–42
Cultural knowledge, 42
Culturally responsive care, 89
Cultural norms, 114
Cultural practices, 40
Cultural sensitivity, 153
Culture, 38, 159
  impact of, 39, 158, 159
  issues, failure to, 39, 40
  tips for, 40, 41

D
Data analysis, 123
Data collection, 123
Data sharing, 78
Depression, 64
  rheumatic condition, 10–12
Digital divide, 139-148
  in rheumatology, 142–144
Digital tools, 75, 78
Dignity, 153
Diverse populations, 156
Doctor-patient communication, 8

E
Electronic health records (EHRs), 75, 78, 132
Electronic medical records (EMRs), 74
Empathy, 22
Engagement, 152
  ingredients for, 153
  multicultural populations, in research, 156, 157
  script, 154, 155
  tips, 154
European League Against Rheumatism (EULAR), 73, 103

F
Family and support systems, 87
  adolescent development, stages of, 93
  Charla de Lupus (Lupus Chat)® Program, 93, 94
  chronic illness and the family experience, 89
  interdisciplinary colleagues, 88
  patient and family advisory councils, 88
  psychosocial support groups, 88
  shared decision-making, 88
Federal Communications Commission (FCC), 142
Fragmented health care delivery system, 75

G
Gender identity, 51
Gender-neutral language, 53
Grief, 3, 4

H
HEADSSS Assessment, 50
Health beliefs, 40
Healthcare organizations, 49
Healthcare providers, 15
Healthcare system factors, 63
Health disparities, 109, 110
  drivers of, 110
  non-medical drivers of health, 111

strategy clinicians, 112
implicit bias, 112–118
Health literacy, 32, 100
and self-management, 99, 100
communication and, 101, 102
LupusLine® Program, 104, 105
National Support and Education Programs, 103, 104
support and education programs, 102, 103
tips for providers, 101
Health-related social needs (HRSNs), 121, 124
Healthy People 2020, 49
Healthy People 2030, 99, 111
Hospital anxiety and depression scale (HADS), 18
Hospital Commitment to Health Equity, 123

I

Implicit association test (IAT), 115
Implicit bias, 44, 112, 159
addressing, 115
client, 114
decision-making process and check for, 116
dignity and respect, practice from, 115, 116
factors, 113
importance of, 113
spirit of curiosity, 116–118
stress and factors, identify sources of, 116
Inflammatory arthritis (IA), 97
Inpatient prospective payment system (IPPS), 122
Inpatient Quality Reporting (IQR) program, 122–123
In-person appointments, preparing for, 147
Institute of Medicine, 49
Interdisciplinary collaboration, 80
Interprofessional team, 2
Intimacy, 7, 8

J

Joint Commission Health Disparities Standard, 123
Joint pain, 92

L

Lesbian, gay, bisexual, transgender, queer/questioning, intersex, asexual, or other sex/gender minorities (LGBTQIA+), 48, 49, 158
direct practice, 52–55
disparities, 50
identity and rheumatology, 50
organizational and macro-level interventions, 55
affirming spaces, 55
community, feedback from, 58
hospital-wide committee, form/join, 55, 56
inclusive policies, 57
sexual orientation and gender identity, 56, 57
staff trainings, 56
system enhancement, 57, 58
research, 49
terms, 51
Linear progression, 4
LupusLine® Program, 104, 105
Lupus nephritis, 90

M

Medication regimens, 65
Mental health, 68, 141, 142
rheumatic condition, 9, 10

Mental health screening, 16, 17
- beck depression inventory, 17
- C-SSRS, 17
- hospital anxiety and depression scale, 18
- PHQ-8 and PHQ9, 17
- PROMIS®, 18

Mindfulness-based practices, 10
Mindfulness-based stress reduction (MBSR), 10
Minimal encouragers, 155
Motivational interviewing, 31
Mutual respect, 80

N

National Culturally and Linguistically Appropriate Services (CLAS), 38
National Institutes of Health, 18
National LGBTQIA+ Health Education Center, 51, 56
National transgender discrimination survey, 49
NIH Minority Health and Health Disparities Strategic Plan 2021-2025, 157
Nonadherence, 61
Non-medical drivers of health, 111

O

Office of the National Coordinator (ONC), 57
Open-ended questions, 156
Organizational health literacy, 100

P

Patient and family advisory councils, 88
Patient care, 87
- adolescent development, stages of, 93
- chronic illness and the family experience, 89
- interdisciplinary colleagues, 88
- patient and family advisory councils, 88
- psychosocial support groups, 88
- shared decision-making, 88

Patient-centered care, 1, 74, 80
Patient-doctor relationship, 4
Patient education, 67, 97
Patient Health Questionnaires Depression scale, 17
- PHQ-8, 17
- PHQ9, 17

Patient journey, 1
Patient participation
- barriers to, 161–163
- in clinical trials and research studies, 151

Patient-provider partnership, 21, 22
- affirmation, 31
- disparities and communication, 26
- doctor's responsibilities, 24, 25
- goals of, 22–24
- motivational interviewing, 31
- open ended questions, 31
- patient's responsibilities, 25, 26
- preparing patients, 28–30
- reflective listening, 31
- responsibilities, 24
- shared decision-making, 27
- summarization, 32
- teach-back method, 32–34
- tools for, 27

Patient-provider relationship, 64, 122, 124
Patient recruitment, to combat bias, 159–161
Patient-related factors, 64–65
Patient Reported Outcomes Measurement Information System (PROMIS®), 18

Patient values
assessments, 43, 44
implicit bias, 44
tips for, 40, 41
Personal health literacy, 99
Physical symptoms, 3
Physician factors, 64
Practice mindful listening, 155
Primary care provider (PCP), 50
Psychological safety, 82
Psycho-social-emotional aspects of care
mental health screening, 16, 17
beck depression inventory, 17
C-SSRS, 17
hospital anxiety and depression scale, 18
PHQ-8 and PHQ9, 17
PROMIS®, 18
risk, assessment and intervention, 15, 16
Psychosocial impact, 2
Psychosocial support groups, 88

R
Readiness, engaging patients for, 152
Reimbursement models, 76
Reproductive health, 50
Respect, 152, 153
Rheumatic condition, 3
depression and anxiety in, 10–12
loss and grief when living with, 3, 4
mental health considerations, 9, 10
navigating work accommodations, 7
relationships and social roles, 5, 6
sex and intimacy, 7–9
Rheumatic disease, 50, 87, 98
Rheumatic illness, 1, 73
Rheumatoid arthritis (RA), 7
Rheumatology, 121, 135
COVID-19 on, 139, 140
rheumatology specialty hospital study, 140–142
providers, 80
telehealth and digital divide in, 142–144

S
Safety, 152
Self-efficacy, 98, 99
Self-management, 97–99
goals of, 97
health literacy and, 99, 100
communication and, 101, 102
LupusLine®Program, 104, 105
national support and education programs, 103, 104
support and education programs, 102, 103
tips for providers, 101
strategies, use of, 98
Sex, 7, 8
Sex assigned at birth, 51
Sexual dysfunction, 8
Sexual orientation and gender identity (SOGI), 56, 57
SHARE approach, 27, 28
Shared decision-making, 27, 88
Shared savings programs, 78
Siloed healthcare delivery system, 75
Social determinants of health (SDOH), 68, 111, 121
implementing screening, 124
direct practice, 124
social history, 125–137
standardized organization-wide collection, 127–134
regulatory guidance, 122, 123
Socioeconomic factors, 62–63

Staff training, 56
Standardized organization-wide collection
  collection, workflow design for, 129, 130
  documentation and information sharing, 133, 134
  electronic health record, 132, 133
  interdisciplinary workgroup, assembling, 127, 128
  intervention, workflow design for, 130–132
  reporting and evaluation, 134
  screening tool, identifying, 128, 129
  training and communication, 133
Substance Abuse and Mental Health Services (SAMHSA), 54
Suicide risk, 15
Systemic lupus erythematosus (SLE), 3

T
Teach-back method, 32–34, 118, 155
Team approach
  psychological safety, 82
  team-based care
    barriers to, 75–77
    optimization, 77–81
Team-based care
  barriers to, 75–77
  optimization, 77–81
Telehealth, 78
  rheumatology, 142–144
Telehealth disparities
  strategies to, 145
    in-person appointments, preparing for, 147
    preparing for appointments, 146
    telehealth/telemedicine tip sheet, 145
    telemedicine appointments, preparing for, 146, 147
Telemedicine, 140
Therapeutic alliance, 2
Therapeutic relationships, 22
Therapy-related factors, 65, 66
Transgender, 51
Transportation, 81
Trauma-informed care, 54
Trust, 152

U
Uncertainty, 3
Unpredictability, 3

V
Value-based payment models, 78

W
World Health Organization (WHO), 61, 62

Z
Z codes, 133

The manufacturer's authorised representative in the EU is Springer Nature Customer Service Centre GmbH, Europaplatz 3, 69115 Heidelberg, Germany. If you have any concerns regarding our products, please contact ProductSafety@springernature.com

Printed and bound by CPI Group (UK) Ltd, Croydon, CR0 4YY
30/09/2026
02225474-0001